Practising Public Health

An Eyewitness Account

Practising
Public Health
An Eyewitness Account

John Ashton

Foreword by

Liam J. Donaldson

To Alan + Alex + Sacha!
(and Dora + Harold)
with immense love.
John.
December 2019.

OXFORD
UNIVERSITY PRESS

OXFORD

UNIVERSITY PRESS

Great Clarendon Street, Oxford, OX2 6DP,
United Kingdom

Oxford University Press is a department of the University of Oxford.
It furthers the University's objective of excellence in research, scholarship,
and education by publishing worldwide. Oxford is a registered trade mark of
Oxford University Press in the UK and in certain other countries

Published in the United States of America by Oxford University Press
198 Madison Avenue, New York, NY 10016, United States of America

British Library Cataloguing in Publication Data

Data available

Library of Congress Control Number: 2019949849

ISBN 978–0–19–874317–0

Printed and bound by
CPI Group (UK) Ltd, Croydon, CR0 4YY

Foreword

A number of years ago, I was browsing in a record shop in Newcastle upon Tyne. It was in the dying days of the CD and at the breaking dawn of the MP3 era; no sign at that point of a vinyl revival. I was buying the latest release by Bob Dylan and remarking to the shop's owner what a lambasting it had received from the critics.

I had found him to be a man of few words but worth listening to for musical recommendations. As he handed me my change he said simply: "Yes, but he's done it all, hasn't he? God bless him."

When I had finished reading the final draft of John Ashton's book, that comment popped into my mind. Perhaps it was a cosmic connection that put it there. John lived in Newcastle when he was at the university's medical school as an undergraduate. I spent 12 happy years there as Regional Director of Public Health. And we are both inveterate Bob Dylan fans.

The power and rugged character of two mighty northern rivers—the Tyne and the Mersey—cannot have failed to stir John's interest in place, regional identity, and history. All three are woven into the accounts of the life and times captured in a fascinating series of chapters that scope the breadth and depth of modern public health.

These two northern territories of the public health landscape of England also serve as a strategic and moral compass for practitioners even today. They are characterized by the depth of the pockets of deprivation, the scale of health inequalities, the missed opportunities for health, and the devastating consequences of an adverse early life experience. As shines through in the pages of this book, such priorities fired John at the start of his career, drove him on, and still ignite his passion even today.

The range of practical initiatives that John created and led in the North West during his time as a public health professor at Liverpool University and then Regional Director of Public Health is formidable. This was not just in population health but improvements to the NHS too. John spanned academic and service public health in an exemplary way and describes his approach. He quotes the late Geoffrey Rose whom he knew from his time at the London School of Hygiene and Tropical Medicine who said that public health practitioners should have "Clean minds and dirty hands."

Public health history is an interest of many but, throughout his career, John has been quite unique in the way that he has linked past events and major historical figures to the challenges of the day. There are many points in the book where the voices of the early medical officers of health and the Victorian sanitary reformers seem to echo at every turn.

Strongest amongst them is William Henry Duncan (1805–63), Liverpool's and the country's first Medical Officer of Health; John leaves us in no doubt about his legacy and honours it in his own work in Liverpool. He describes how, at a dark time in the city's history, he sought to bring transformative health regeneration. He used *Esmedune*, the Saxon name for the Toxteth area of the city where there had been major riots, as a politically neutral word, to launch a future city initiative intended to facilitate a fresh and optimistic approach to apparently intractable problems. He links back again to history when citing the inspiration of artist, designer, and social activist William Morris's (1834–96) utopian vision of a harmonious and balanced city.

The city-focused public health programmes in Liverpool became a model for the highly innovative World Health Organization *Healthy Cities* initiative. John was one of the principal architects of this. It started in 1986 and is continuing over 30 years later. It has benefitted the health and environment of tens of millions of citizens of cities across the world. John describes the process of bringing people together, gaining commitment, and negotiating the political hurdles.

Those who have seen John in full flow at meetings or at conference podia, powerful and charismatic, will be fascinated by the sections of the book that describe those who have shaped him as a person and a public health leader. There are many and he speaks of his mentors with great reverence and humility.

Three-quarters of the way through the book, I put it down to make a cup of coffee and thought: '*I cannot imagine anyone else who could have written this.*'

It is part poignant memoir, part history lesson, part manifesto for health, part paean for a fairer society, part portfolio of practical case studies, part handbook for local, national, and global public health leadership, and part letter to a future generation.

Indeed, he has done it all. This wonderful book was a joy and an inspiration to read.

Liam J. Donaldson
Chief Medical Officer for England (1998–2010)

Preface

It is the best of times and the worst of times for public health. On the one hand, we have never had such a strong, evidence-based position from which to tackle the scourges that impact on the human condition and human populations. But on the other hand, living in an increasingly globalized and complex economic, environmental, and social system, the fragility of our situation and the capacity of humans to soil their own nest has never been more apparent. New threats are constantly appearing, whether from climate change, war, conflict, and population displacement, or from the emergence of new infectious diseases and increasing importance of long-term conditions.

In parallel, public health has become much more prominent in recent years, as a casual perusal of the media will testify, but we still have great difficulty in mobilizing the organized efforts of society to protect and improve health in a timely way. The anti-health forces often seem to hold most of the cards. Our capacity for advocacy and political action often seem weak and our institutions of government not fit for purpose when it comes to public health. Too often we are driving using the rear-view mirror. The international United Nations Agencies, including the World Health Organization, which were established in the aftermath of the Second World War, to protect against the preconditions for conflict, can be caught off-guard, as happened with Ebola in west Africa.

There has been a growing body of knowledge over the past 30 years about how best to intervene at a population level to secure good health and wellbeing. The importance of whole systems intervention through multi- and interdisciplinary efforts has increasingly been recognized and there has been an explosion of education courses. There has also been a rapid growth of online global options for public health study, but there is a shortage of contemporary, suitable texts that link theory to practice and transaction to transformation with actual case studies. There is an abundance of epidemiological and statistical textbooks but remarkably few that share the experience of actually 'doing public health'. This book is an attempt to at least partially fill that gap. It builds on the earlier publication of *The New Public Health*, which I wrote with my colleague Howard Seymour when we were both starting our practical journey. Since then I have much more to report.

As a public health doctor, I had a wide clinical background before entering public health in the 1980s. I have also worked extensively in public health academia and the world of public health practice; I have always tried to bridge the two. I believe that my public health education proper only began when I first met and became involved with the Vauxhall community in north Liverpool—they taught me much of what I know about co-production and authentic public health transformation. I will retell that story here and will also draw on a wide range of interventions which I, and others, have been involved with since that time.

Although in one sense this is a parochial and personal account, in another it drills up to the national and international levels to capture the 'strategic under view'. This reflects my experience as one who has been privileged to work in the different theatres and population aggregates that public health must address. Examples will include illustrations from a 'total place' or 'settings' approach, Community-Orientated Primary Care, and Asset-Based Community Development. The philosophy of the book, to quote the late Professor Geoffrey Rose of the London School of Hygiene and Tropical Medicine, is that to make a difference in public health it is necessary to have 'a clean mind and dirty hands', and that research and teaching should go hand in glove with public participation. I hope that the reader finds it worthwhile.

John Ashton, September 2019

Acknowledgements

How do you begin to pay proper tribute to all those who have shaped and had a hand in over 40 years' work and a joyous adventure that continues as I write? This story covers a journey that encompasses five continents and many cities, has taken place during two marriages with three families, six children, and some amazing people.

As the youngest child of an unconditionally supportive family I was part of the much blessed post-Second World War cohort of baby boomers born in the heady years of demobilization and the desire to build a better, peaceful future. I had no silver spoon in my mouth but an abundance of maternal care, Welfare Orange, National Dried Milk, and the benefits of a welfare state which aimed to do its best for all of us. With an insulin-dependent father in humble employment, none of my journey would have been likely without the Beveridge Report of 1942, the Butler Education Act of 1944, or the single mindedness of Nye Bevan and the post-war Labour government.

Every step of the way I found mentors and supporters, who gave selflessly, provided guidance, opened my mind and with it many doors. At Newstead Farm in Woolton and in South Liverpool, I acquired a confidence that came with responsibility. At Quarry Bank High School in Liverpool, sometime Eton of the Labour Party, my political and social awareness was prompted by John Ashcroft and headmaster Bill Pobjoy offered me self-belief; he was to continue sending me notes of support in my public life until his death almost 50 years later. Dora and Harold Hayling, my back-up parents, built on my quest for social justice with continuing political education, internationalism, and insights into developmental and educational psychology which have followed me through life. In Newcastle in the 1960s the medical school under a succession of remarkable deans was undergoing a student-centred revolution which straddled the incredible year of 1968, when it was such a joy to be alive and to become 21 years old. John Walker, Andrew Smith, and Donald Irvine showed me public health and family medicine; Christine Cooper and Donald Court showed me community child health; Martin Roth and a team to rival anything from London sparked my interest in mental health; and Mary Peberdy kindled a lifelong interest in sexual health and planned parenthood. It was a breathlessly formative time. And it was also the time that I met my first wife, Pam, who was to share my life for almost 30 years with Keir, Matt, and Nick, as we explored together how best to contribute to the organized efforts of society for health and wellbeing.

Once I had joined the ranks of public health workers there were many more supporters and guides who paved the way and provided encouragement, many of them mentioned in these pages—Jerry Morris, Sidney Chave, and Bob Logan at the London School of Hygiene and Tropical Medicine; Bryan Abel Smith, John Carrier, Jenny Roberts, and others at the London School of Economics; Donald Acheson (another writer of notes), William McKee, John Revans, and John Dennis in Southampton and Wessex; and afterwards Tom Hobday, Donald Wilson, Duncan Nichol, Ruth Hussey, Julie Hotchkiss, Mark Bellis, Adrian Henri, Catherine Marcangeli, Fred O'Brien, Rob Mcdonald, Bill Halsall, Tony McGann, the people of the Vauxhall neighbourhood, and a plethora of colleagues and friends in Liverpool and the North West, who together built something very special and enduring. Together with Howard Seymour we lit a spark. In Cumbria our amazing team included Sue Page, Mike Taylor, Mike Bewick, Moira Angel, Irving Cobden, Neela Shabde, Mark Graham, and Ross Forbes.

In Parliament and London too, I was most fortunate with collaboration and support from politicians and public servants including Julia Cumberlege, Tessa Jowell, Philip Hunt, Nigel Crisp, and most recently Sarah Wollaston. In the three years of my presidency of the UK Faculty of Public Health, David Allen, Jane Dacre, and a squad of college presidents were generous in their unconditional support even when I didn't make it easy. B. Sethia as President of the Royal Society of Medicine was an anchor when I needed it.

For the past 20 years my journey has been with my second wife and constant companion, Maggi, and has included her two sons Alex (Sandy) and Dylan, and our own late lamb, Che. Having family members from each decade of life has kept me more grounded than would have otherwise been the case and Maggi has brought me back constantly to the schism of C. P. Snow's two cultures, having herself made the remarkable transition from anthropology and art history to become a Director of Public Health; an additional bonus being to know her father Terence Morris, LSE pioneer of post-war criminology.

One of the joys of work in public health is the never-ending prospect of meeting new influences, most recently Anthony Seldon, and renewing old. The WHO Healthy Cities strand has lasted over 30 years so far and includes Ilona Kickbusch, Trevor Hancock, Chris Gates, Rodrigo Guerrero, Alberto Concha Eastman, Evelyne De Leeuw, and many others. I met our mentor Lowell Levin and Corinne and Joanna through WHO, a profound and enduring relationship; and fellow American John McKnight, the father of Asset-Based Community Development and his wife, Marsha, have become close friends. As I write

I have the huge privilege of working with Monika Kosinska, who now leads Healthy Cities for WHO together with Adam Tiliouine, and am immersed with Trevor and Evelyne with Ada Brunstein at Oxford University Press in the ambitious project of a global encyclopaedia of Healthy Cities and Communities. In 2018–19, Maggi and I were humbled to work with the communities of North Kensington and those affected by the tragedy of the Grenfell Tower Disaster, supported by Chief Executive Barry Quirk and Cabinet Member for Health David Lindsay and currently life has come full circle as I work as public health adviser to the Right Honorable Jane Kennedy, Police and Crime Commissioner for Merseyside on the challenging agenda of applying a public health approach to the prevention of violence.

This book would never have seen the light of day without the belief and support of Maggi. I hope that readers will feel it has been worth the effort. Thank you everybody.

Contents

Part I

On the shoulders of giants

Chapter 1

Roots and foundations

'The health of the people is the highest law' (1) proclaims the plaque to be found above the doorway of Southwark Town Hall in South London. This text was originally taken from Cicero's *De Legibus*, contained in Bentham's book of quotations in 1948.

That a London borough council should have cited Cicero as its overarching mission statement in the first half of the twentieth century was no accident. Concerns about population health go back at least 2,000 years, with references to the laws for healthy living to be found in the Bible and other historic texts. Many Old Testament proverbs provide guidance on how to live a full and healthy life. The Victorian public health movement, which provides a backcloth to this book, was very much rooted in the town hall—a democratic institution with its elected members accountable directly to the local citizens.

From the earliest days a tension has existed between prevention and treatment and care. In Greek mythology Aesculapius, the god of medicine, had two daughters, Hygieia and Panacea. For the worshippers of Hygieia, health was the natural order of things, a positive attribute to which people were entitled if they governed their lives wisely. The followers of Panacea, more skeptically, believed that the chief role of the physician was to treat disease and restore health. This was to be done by correcting imperfections caused by the accidents of birth and life, and to restore disturbances in the balance of equilibrium between the elements constituting the human body.

The Romans too were most concerned about public health and hygiene and not least about sanitation. The remains of the remarkable Roman sanitary engineering are still to be seen as far as the outer fringes of the Roman Empire. But somehow much of the empirical knowledge of these ancient times seems to have been eclipsed in subsequent centuries and by the time of the Industrial Revolution and the rapid urbanization that accompanied it, hard lessons had to be learned all over again. For example, Roman egg-shaped sewers found in parts of Italy were rediscovered in Liverpool in the 1840s when the local borough engineer transformed the sanitary condition of the slum areas by constructing many miles of them.

In the United Kingdom, the 'rise of the Public Health Movement' began with the Great Reform Act of 1832, in the aftermath of the Napoleonic Wars. Major challenges were posed to public health by the movement of large numbers of people from the rural areas to the booming industrial cities of the north of England, and by the slum conditions created in their wake. On the political front the 1832 Great Reform Act did away with rotten boroughs, distributed parliamentary seats on a population basis, and gave the vote to £10 householders. It began the long journey to modern democracy and citizen empowerment. This was reinforced by the Municipal Corporations Act, which extended the vote to taxpayers outside London. Of more immediate relevance to public health was the Poor Law Amendment Act of 1834, which amended the 1601 Poor Law Act and tackled the problems created by the enclosure of common land and the creation of beggars, by making parishes responsible for the care of their own poor.

This 'public health movement' gathered momentum in 1832 and 1837 when cholera first made an unwelcome appearance in the slums of Europe. Anybody studying public health in London today will have had an early acquaintance with the story of John Snow and the Broad Street pump. It is through such stories that public health is brought to life, lessons are best learned, and the baton is passed on from generation to generation.

The story of John Snow actually predates Soho and London and begins in Newcastle upon Tyne where John Snow was apprenticed at the age of 14 to a local surgeon, William Hardcastle. This was at the time when cholera was first making an appearance in Sunderland in 1831, carried from the outer reaches of the Empire by the merchant fleet. It was to arouse this young man's curiosity when he later had the chance to act on an insight of huge importance during the 1854 cholera epidemic in Soho. If serendipity is said to favour the prepared mind, then John Snow's mind was prepared as a tender youth on Tyneside. Such curiosity is surely the very bedrock of effective public health practice.

By the time he found himself in Broad Street Market in 1854, Snow was making a reputation for himself by administering chloroform anaesthesia to Queen Victoria in her last two confinements (Leopold in 1853, and later Beatrice in 1857); this in defiance of the pope who had ruled that childbirth was supposed to be painful. Clearly no shrinking violet, he opened the way for millions of women to have a better experience of childbirth and in so doing taught us the importance of standing up to authority and dogma in the interests of the public health.

The 1854 cholera outbreak was focused around Broad Street in Soho beginning in August with the death of a baby, at 40 Broad Street, from 'exhaustion following sickness and diarrhoea'. This child's illness immediately preceded the onset of the epidemic which built up to a peak of 56 total cases between 31

August and 2 September. Snow's curiosity being aroused, he set about collecting data on the deaths in partnership with the Reverend Henry Whitehead of St Luke's parish in Berwick Street and Dr Edwin Lankester, soon to become the first Medical Officer of Health to St James's.

Whitehead discovered that the faeces of the baby who had died had been disposed of in a cesspit less than three feet from the well. A major contrast was between the numbers of deaths in the Eley percussion cap factory where there were 14 deaths from a workforce of 20 and the local brewery where there were no deaths among the 100 workmen. That the men in the brewery had access to water from a deep well was strong supportive evidence for the water from the street pump being responsible. Additional support came from Professor Frankland of the Royal College of Chemistry who used dyes to demonstrate diffusion from a cesspit adjacent to the pump where local mothers steeped their infants' nappies. However, with the dominant theory of contagion being that of the 'miasma' or bad air (this being some years before the Pasteurs came up with the germ theory of disease), Snow had a battle on his hands. He needed to persuade the local select church vestry who were responsible for the street pump to remove the handle and disable it. The clinching evidence came from Snow making the trip to Hampstead to investigate the one outlying death that turned out to be Mrs Eley, the widow of the owner of the percussion cap factory. Having grown up in the neighbourhood, Mrs Eley was so fond of the water from the pump, which was clear, bright, and sparkling, that she had bottles of the well water brought to her by cart. Armed with this information Snow was able to have the pump handle removed on Friday 8th September. Ironically, by this time the epidemic had already peaked but Snow gained the credit and celebrity status for ending the epidemic.

There are many lessons in the life and work of John Snow but the importance of shoe leather epidemiology and of teamwork are timeless, as too is the robust way in which he challenged the orthodoxy of the day. That John Snow has such a hallowed place in the tradition of public health is perhaps not surprising given that he was operating on the metropolitan canvass with a high profile and highly feared outbreak. Years later we were to see much the same kind of issue arise with regard to who was recognized in the battle against HIV/AIDS.

While John Snow was making his name in London, William Henry Duncan, a Liverpolitan of Scottish extraction, was making his mark in Liverpool (see Figure 1.1). When Edwin Chadwick—one of the principal authors of the Poor Law Report of 1832—was soliciting information on the health of slum dwellers in the industrial cities, local Liverpool doctor Duncan responded enthusiastically.

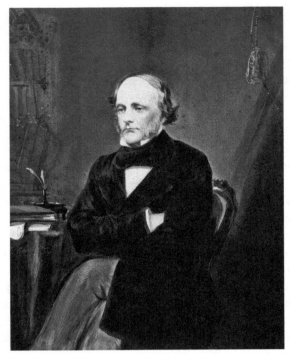

Figure 1.1 Dr William Henry Duncan, 1805–63, England's First Medical Officer of Health.
Reproduced with permission from Ian F. L. Duncan.

Edwin Chadwick had been appointed to be the first Poor Law Commissioner, having come under the influence of Jeremy Bentham, the great utilitarian philosopher. His philosophy of always seeking the greatest good for the greatest number was seen as the test of any policy and a thread of this can be seen to run through health policy from that time. As Bentham's research assistant, Chadwick had seen the close connection between disease and poverty and he loathed waste. A lawyer by training, he always wanted facts, employing three doctors as investigators who visited the manufacturing towns, took evidence, and wrote reports.

Duncan's evidence was influential with Chadwick and contributed to Chadwick's 1842 report on the 'Sanitary Condition of the Labouring Population'. This was a damning indictment of the conditions of the working class in industrial towns and led to the development of 'the sanitary idea' as a theory of causation and as a methodology and set of administrative arrangements for dealing with it.

Duncan developed Chadwick's theme locally in papers and talks given to the Literary and Philosophical Society of Liverpool. With regard to cellars in 1844, he wrote, 'The cellars are ten or twelve feet square; generally flagged—but frequently having only the bare earth for a floor, and sometimes less than six feet in height. There is frequently no window; so that light and air can gain access to the room only by the door, the top of which is often not higher than the street' (2). Based on his lectures, Duncan published a pamphlet entitled 'The Physical Causes of the High Rate of Mortality in Liverpool', in which he demonstrated that the average age of death in the counties of Rutland and Wiltshire was 36½ years, compared with 19 years in Liverpool, Manchester, Leeds, and Bolton. Duncan's high profile advocacy, his careful choice of hard-hitting statistics, and his vivid descriptions were influential in persuading the town council to promote a private Bill in Parliament which came to be the Liverpool 'Sanatory' (*sic*) Act of 1846.

The Liverpool Sanatory Act was groundbreaking in that it picked up a proposal from Chadwick's *Report* and made it happen. 'That for the general promotion of the means necessary to prevent disease it would be good economy to appoint a district medical officer independent of private practice, and with the securities of special qualifications and responsibilities to initiate sanitary measures, and reclaim the execution of the law' (3). The Liverpool Act detailed a job description for such a position including regular inspection and reporting on diseases, epidemics, and nuisances, and advice on the measures to be taken to check or prevent the spread of disease. The act also gave the borough powers over street paving and restriction of the construction of the narrow court type of housing which appeared to be incriminated in creating the types of housing conducive to slums and epidemics, as well as an obligation to sewer and drain the borough.

This Liverpool Act paved the way for the appointment not only of a Medical Officer of Health but also for a 'qualified Civil Engineer to act as Local Surveyor' and an 'Inspector of Nuisances', all to work under the Health Committee of the town council. This Liverpool Act influenced the drafting of the Public Health Act of 1848, the appointment of a Medical Officer of Health (MOH) for the City of London the following year and of MOsH in many other local authorities subsequently.

Duncan's appointment as Medical Officer of Health for Liverpool was not in doubt and it was confirmed by the Secretary of State as required by the Liverpool Act on 1 January 1847. This was not a moment too soon.

Slum dwelling and the rise of the public health movement

The story of the work of Dr Duncan and his colleagues in Liverpool is a rich one which captures the rise of Liverpool as the major port of the British Empire, drawing in the displaced masses from the north of England to create the world's first large-scale urban slums.

According to Duncan's biographer, Frazer, the main emphasis of public health work until the twentieth century was on sanitation, made necessary by the appalling squalor of the hastily thrown-up slum housing. The focus was on managing and controlling outbreaks of infectious disease through action on its predisposing environmental causes—the housing itself, the 'nuisances' (especially human, animal, and vegetable waste, which was to be found everywhere), the inspection of food, together with efforts to improve the conditions to be found in the myriad of low grade and overcrowded lodging houses. This first phase of 'modern' (nineteenth-century) public health, with its environmental focus, centred on the need to separate human and animal waste from food and water, the so-called 'sanitary idea'. All actions stemmed from this imperative and all occurred in the absence of a robust, evidence-based knowledge of the biology of infection. Today we would describe this focus as being upstream and on the determinants of health and disease. These early practitioners had had no formal training in epidemiology or population health; rather they came from practical disciplines but had an instinct for the bigger picture. Snow, Duncan, and their contemporaries were at work some twenty years before the Pasteurs put forward the germ theory of disease. Notions of bad air and gases or the miasma generated by rotting matter prevailed. Snow's proposal that the cholera was water borne in Soho in 1854 was met with considerable hostility from some. Meanwhile, in Liverpool Duncan appears to have been an adherent of the miasma theory, believing that the contamination of the atmosphere when people were closely crowded together was contagious and could spread typhus and other fevers, and he began to favour the role of flies as a vector. A water source was not on the agenda in the Liverpool slums and the peak of the cholera outbreaks tended to correspond to the summer peaks of the fly populations.

Duncan's collaboration with Chadwick extended beyond his report, 'The Condition of The Poor', to the evidence that he gave before a Select Committee of the House of Commons. According to Frazer, Duncan's 'sympathies with the poor and interest in sanitary reform enhanced the value of his services when they were placed at the disposal of the borough and enabled him to endure the inevitable failures of the pioneer and the opprobrium which has always been the fate of the reformer' (4). At this time, local centres of population, such as the emerging industrial cities of the north of England, had become economic power bases in their own right with a 'race of merchant princes' riding high on a wave of commerce with the colonies. Viewed from the twenty-first century where incessant centralization has led to an emasculation of local government, it is difficult to conjure up the sense of autonomy that must have driven these early pioneers. For Frazer, 'the work of those at the centre was important, but all the recommendations of the various commissions on the health of the labouring classes would have been useless if they had not been brought into effect at the periphery by the devoted labours of sanitary pioneers in the larger towns in the middle years of the last century' (4).

It is in this context and against today's debates about devolution of powers that we might consider the real scope for a city such as Liverpool to take concerted action and take control of its own public health destiny. Until the Municipal Corporations Act of 1835, Liverpool had been governed by a self-elected body but after 1835 an 'energetic (Whig) reforming council ... began vigorously to deal with police, sanitation, lighting and cleansing' (4). The upshot in terms of a legislative framework was the Liverpool Building Act of 1842 which made the building of narrow courts unlawful, the Liverpool Improvement Act of the same year which strengthened the governance of the police and put in place meat and slaughterhouse inspection, and most importantly the Liverpool Sanatory Act of 1846, which led to Duncan's appointment as Medical Officer of Health. A health committee held all three areas to account.

Meanwhile, the publication of Chadwick's report in 1842 had provided an energizing focus of its own. One immediate outcome was the appearance in 1844 of the Health of Towns Association with branches around the country. This was a body which would come to play an important part in pressurising the government into sanitary reform. The historian Finer cites a number of voluntary associations which came into being around 1844, including the Association for Promoting Cleanliness among the Poor (aiming to set up baths and wash houses), and the Society for the Improvement of the Conditions of the Labouring Classes (aimed at providing model dwellings for rent). The Health of Towns Association was formed at a public meeting in Exeter Hall on the Strand in London on 11th December. Finer describes it as an 'avowed propagandist body ... of capital importance' (5). At this first meeting it was stated that the association was formed with the purpose of sharing information gained from recent inquiries made into the terrible living conditions of much of the population. The aim was to assist changes in the law that would allow for improvement to be carried out by preparing the public for such changes.

Following the first meeting of the national Health of Towns Association in December 1844, branches were quickly formed in Edinburgh, Liverpool,

Manchester, York, Halifax, Derby, Bath, Rugby, Marlborough, Walsall, Plymouth, and Worcester. The local bodies worked by disseminating facts and figures drawn from official reports; by organizing public lectures on the subject; by reporting on the sanitary problems of their district; and by organizing public meetings to petition parliament. The public lectures instructed audiences of both the working and middle classes in the elementary principles of ventilation, drainage, and civic and domestic cleanliness. It was thought that only by pressure from without could changes in the law be affected. If people were aware of how much harm their poor living conditions were causing them, they might be inclined to help press for reform.

In Liverpool the mayor convened a meeting in April 1845, in the music hall in Bold Street, to form a Liverpool branch of the Health of Towns Association. A feature in the *Liverpool Mercury* describes the attendance at this first meeting as being 'not large, but highly respectable', including leading members of the council and both Protestant and Catholic clergymen. In addition to Dr Duncan and his collaborator Dr Samuel Holme, several other members of the medical profession were in attendance. The *Mercury* described those present as 'gentlemen of all sects of religion, and all parties of politics' (4). This meeting passed unanimous resolutions defining the sanitary objects to be aimed at, and called for legislative action. The duty of the association should be to 'collect funds, to supply information, and to furnish those details which must be the basis of all legislation' (4). The meeting set up a local committee which published a monthly journal called the *Liverpool Health of Towns Advocate* for nearly two years, 1,500 copies of the first number being distributed free of charge.

The working class does not appear to have been well represented in the Liverpool association; yet, they were the worst sufferers from the unsanitary conditions. Nevertheless, the association did undoubtedly give good service in obtaining local publicity for the mass of information that was now available on the subject of the massive health inequalities that prevailed. Up until this time many commentators had been under the impression that Liverpool was one of the healthiest towns in the country. This misperception is commonly found in the burgeoning mega cities of the developing world today.

In 1840s Liverpool, the evidence shocked many into calling for action by appealing not only to their civic pride and humanitarianism, but also to their self-interest. The evidence demonstrated that whilst the poor suffered the worst, they were not the only ones to suffer and there was in fact a gradient. The gentry in Liverpool were shown to have worse mortality rates than the gentry in Leeds and London. Local activist Samuel Holme, at the first meeting of the Liverpool association and as reported in the *Liverpool Mercury*, suggested that 'in endeavouring to ameliorate the conditions of the lower classes ... They would benefit themselves, for they were all breathing in the same polluted atmosphere' (4). Such observations have resonances in contemporary writing on inequalities in health, for example in the *Spirit Level* by Richard Wilkinson and Kate Pickett and the work of Sir Michael Marmot.

At the same meeting Dr Duncan quoted statistics for the average age of death in Liverpool, taken from the parochial registers of St Nicholas church. During 1784–1810 the average age at death of tradesmen was 23½ and of operatives 18½. By 1841–2 the average age at death of tradesmen had fallen to 19 and for operatives to 16. He also quotes figures for the Moorfields schools where 'on the average $3^{3}/_{10}$ per cent of the scholars residing in houses were always absent from sickness but that 27 per cent of those residing in cellars were absent from the same cause' (4).

The growth of the Liverpool Health of Towns Association led to other bodies becoming concerned about public health. One such body was the Liverpool Guardian Society for the Protection of Trade. They conducted an inquiry in 1845 into Liverpool's water supply. According to White, they concluded that not only was the Liverpool water supply miserably inadequate, but it was almost the most expensive in the country. Suspicions were expressed that the supply was deliberately restricted to keep up monopoly profits and the suggestion was made that the supply would be better if unified under a public authority.

Meanwhile, in London the Metropolitan Working Classes' Association for Improving the Public Health was organized with the motto 'We can be useful no longer than we are well' and in Newcastle and Gateshead a Working Men's Association was formed in alliance with the local Sanitary Association and similar associations were set up in many other towns. The galvanizing impact of Chadwick's report and widespread local action generated a remarkable momentum for sanitary reform. This came not a moment too soon in the face of recurring outbreaks and epidemics and not least with the impending crisis of the potato famine in Ireland.

The Irish potato famine, the 1849 cholera epidemic, and the work of Duncan, Newlands, and Fresh in Liverpool

Duncan's appointment as Medical Officer of Health in 1847 coincided with what Frazer describes as 'two calamitous years' for Liverpool, occasioned by the devastating impact of the Irish potato famine on Irish peasants and their mass flight from starvation. The famine began in 1845, caused by the spread of a fungal infection, *Phytophthora infestans*, in this staple food of a large part of the Irish population. The flight reached massive proportions in 1846–7, when as described by Duncan in his first public health report:

> The 1st of January 1847 found this pauper immigration steadily increasing, and it continued in such rapidly progressively rates, that by the end of June not less than 300,000 Irish had landed in Liverpool. Of these it was very moderately estimated that some 60,000 had located themselves amongst us, occupying every nook and cranny of the already overcrowded lodging houses, and forcing their way into the cellars (about 3,000 in number) which has been closed under the provisions of the Health Act 1842. In different parts of Liverpool 50 or 60 of these destitute people were found in a house containing three or four small rooms, about 12 feet by 10; and in more than one instance upwards of 40 were found sleeping in a cellar. (4)

Over the past few years millions of refugees from civil war in Syria and elsewhere have tried to find sanctuary in Europe. The sense of emergency in Liverpool in 1847 must have been similar and the 1849 cholera epidemic was on its way.

When the cholera returned to Liverpool in 1848–9 it was against a backdrop of what at that time was known as fever or Irish famine fever. This was probably typhus and typhoid with 4–5,000 cases at any one time, necessitating the opening of temporary hospitals and the conversion of lazarettos. In fact, there were three epidemics in progress in 1848, for in addition to fever, scarlatina, and influenza were also doing the rounds. The cholera arrived in Liverpool in December in a court in Back Portland Street where the first victim was a 14-year-old girl. The epidemic peaked the following August and by the time it had finished it had killed 5,245 people in a population of 300,000. In comparison, the 2014 Ebola outbreak in Sierra Leone led to the death of 3,955 people, including 250 health care workers, in a population of six million.

It is likely that the appointment of Duncan as Medical Officer of Health and his action, together with sanitary inspector Thomas Fresh and engineer James Newlands, prevented an altogether worse disaster. The filth and overcrowding had begun to be tackled, extensive whitewashing of courts carried out, temporary hospitals opened, and a system of lay health workers deployed to houses to diagnose and isolate cases. All this in ignorance of the true nature of cholera infection.

Nationally the momentum for government action was building and being fed by experiences such as those from Liverpool. In 1848, the first Public Health Act was passed, a watered-down version of Chadwick's recommendations. The Act permitted local Boards of Health to be established if 10 per cent of ratepayers petitioned for them, unless the crude death rate was 23/1000 or more when a board would be required. The Act also empowered local boards to follow Liverpool's lead and appoint a Medical Officer of Health if they so wished.

By the time of the 1854 cholera epidemic there was the beginning of a body of knowledge relating to public health practice, although it was to be some time before formal university courses would be developed. While Snow was mobilizing his own local co-investigators in Soho, Duncan in Liverpool was determined not to be taken by surprise, as he was in 1849. Then he had repeatedly pressed the Select Vestry to provide hospital accommodation for at least a proportion of the large number of cases of cholera which were occurring. From Frazer's account it is clear that Duncan's relationship with the Vestry was not an easy one and his letter books convey a sense of his frustrations, but his ambitions appear to have prevailed for lime washing to take place and lay health workers to be deployed. When the epidemic was over the death total of 1,146 was considerably less than in 1849 and compares with the Broad Street tally of some 600 in the same year.

The 1854 epidemic and an outbreak in 1866 were the last serious cholera episodes in Liverpool and the measures taken under the legislative provisions of the 1840s appear to have been of importance. Between 1846 and 1866 there had been a considerable reduction in the number of occupied cellar dwellings and much increased supervision of lodging houses. Sanitation, cleanliness, scavenging, street paving, safe water supplies, and street washing had all been put in place. Between 1847 and 1858, Newlands, the engineer, had overseen the construction of 80 miles of sewers, prioritizing areas to be sewered first on the basis of mortality and nuisance data provided by his colleagues Duncan and Fresh. So impressed was Chadwick by the brick-lined design that he promoted it nationally, following the Benthamite principle to 'always do the same thing in the same way, choosing the best and always call the same thing by the same name'. It was to be some years before London's Bazalgette could claim the same level of delivery in London. For Sidney Chave, drafting the first Duncan Memorial Lecture for delivery in Liverpool in 1983, he wrote of Duncan: 'He is not only a reality, he is a power in the commonwealth' (2).

Public health in England after the cholera

This story of public health in the first half of the nineteenth century in Britain tells us how local and national figures responded to international threats to health against the backdrop of massive political and economic fallout from the Industrial Revolution and the hangover from the French Revolution and Napoleonic Wars. In modern parlance it was a whole system story and other countries had their own stories to tell. In Germany and Europe, for example, 1848 came to be known as the 'year of revolution', fuelled in part by these mega trends but also by the process of rapid urbanization and the growth of political movements, not least among the young men arriving in cities from rural areas. The democratization of local government and the vigorous response to threats such as the cholera in some British cities were in the same vein. However, it was not the same everywhere.

Although the 1848 Public Health Act was an important landmark, and despite encouragement by Chadwick, very few local authorities saw fit to appoint Medical Officers of Health. Rather they saw them as an expensive luxury they could afford to do without and by 1853 only 35 are known to have been appointed. In the case of Liverpool, Duncan was initially paid £300 per annum with the right to private practice. However, after an especially sarcastic and critical satire in *Punch* magazine which pointed out the potential conflict of interest inherent in this arrangement, the Council changed his contract to £750 per annum, 'it being understood that he is to give up all private practice and to devote the whole of his time and attention to the duties of the said office' (2).

It would, in fact, take two further Public Health Acts in 1872 and 1875 before each district in the country was required to appoint a Medical Officer of Health—a total of 1,400 in all. Until that time the position of these officers was often precarious and they could be dispensed with if they produced evidence on the public health that was challenging or uncomfortable for the council; it took until 1922 before a Medical Officer of Health could not be dismissed without the consent of a minister and 1929 before Parliament ruled that all appointments were to be full time.

As with security of tenure, so with the independence of public health reports; this was something that was fiercely fought for and established in the ensuing decades.

From sanitation to hygiene and therapy—three eras of public health

A theme that continued to play through the nineteenth century was the tension between local and national action. This was encapsulated by one man in the person of John Simon (pronounced Simone), a surgeon who had been the first Medical Officer of Health to be appointed after Duncan—for the City of London. Simon had effected a sanitary revolution in the city and set a seal of authority on the office of Medical Officer of Health. Every Tuesday morning the vital statistics for the previous week were to be on his desk. He went on to become the country's first Chief Medical Officer from 1855 to 1876. While Simon was building the national foundations for an office which remains today, Chadwick was on a course of self-destruction.

Chadwick bullied the local authorities and soon made himself one of the most detested men in the country; using his centralizing powers of the Board of Health, 'he antagonised the ratepayers because all his schemes cost money; the doctors because "you don't need them—you need engineers" and the engineers by his partiality to those who leaned towards him. Worst of all he antagonised *The Times* which would "rather take our chance with the cholera than be bullied into health by Mr Chadwick" ' (6). The House of Commons threw out the extension of the Board of Health and Chadwick never held public office again. A second Board of Health was established in 1855 but it was a shadow of its former self and although it was renewed annually for three years it was then abolished, with its powers and duties transferred to the Privy Council. Simon was appointed Chief Medical Officer, seeing himself as Medical Officer to the nation with responsibility to educate the politicians and the public.

Simon's vision of a strong central public health department underpinned by a locally based service was at the heart of the Public Health Acts of 1872 and 1875. Unfortunately, according to Chave, 'Gladstone's decision to bring together Public Health and the Poor Law was disastrous with public health being subordinated to the destitution authorities with its deterrent philosophy' (2) and such initiatives as occurred came from local Medical Officers of Health. Although Simon's work built on Chadwick's 'Sanitary Idea', with its environmental focus, a combination of new knowledge from biology together with the benefits from environmental measures were heralding a second era of public health based on hygiene and personal prevention.

The advent of household water supplies, together with the mass production of soap by William and James Lever on Merseyside, paved the way for personal hygiene, whilst the breakthroughs by the Pasteurs and others put vaccine production on a scientific basis. At the same time personal services for health and wellbeing were evolving from their environmental roots. Examples of specific initiatives included:

◆ The Health Visitor movement which had begun in Salford in 1862 when a group of middle class women employed 'a good motherly woman to visit the working class to teach mothers';

◆ The first milk depot to provide milk to nursing mothers in St Helen's in 1899;

◆ The Liverpool Society for the Prevention of Cruelty to Children, the first in the country in 1883; and

◆ The Liverpool Child Welfare Association, the first voluntary organization for the care of crippled children, in 1898.

In Liverpool, innovation on the community nursing front was led by local businessman, philanthropist, and later MP William Rathbone in partnership with

Florence Nightingale and Agnes Jones. District nursing was established in 17 districts with training organized out of the Royal Liverpool Infirmary, a model which soon spread around the country.

Such initiatives were often influenced by the work of early sociologists such as that of Charles Booth on working class life in London, and Rowntree's poverty studies in York. This tradition of quantitative and qualitative research can be traced from Booth via Rowntree to Townsend, Black, Morris, Whitehead, and Marmot since the Second World War. It is a tradition which has stimulated similar work to support public health around the world.

An event of particular importance in the development of public health and prevention in this second era in the British context came about as a result of the Boer War in South Africa from 1899 to 1902. Of those men who had volunteered for military service, 40 per cent were deemed to be unfit and were rejected. Concerns were expressed as to how the country could maintain an imperial race and contain Germany, and an interdepartmental committee on 'physical deterioration' was set up by the government to investigate the decline in physical fitness of the nation after 150 years of global empire. A comprehensive programme of action was proposed:

1. A continuing anthropometric survey
2. Registration of stillbirths
3. Studies of infant mortality
4. Centres for maternal instruction
5. Day nurseries
6. Registration and supervision of working pregnant women
7. Free school meals and medical inspection
8. Physical training for children, training in hygiene and mother craft
9. Prohibition of tobacco sales to children
10. Education on the evils of drink
11. Medicals on entry to work
12. Studies of the prevalence and effects of syphilis
13. Extension of the Health Visiting Service.

At the time there were arguments over community versus family responsibilities for health and wellbeing, an echo of contemporary debates about the so-called 'nanny state' but the nation's interests prevailed and an early outcome was the establishment of a School Meals Service in 1906 and a School Medical Service in 1907. There was compulsory, universal inspection of all children and a system for child health established which spanned government and prevailed until 1974. Modern medicine had yet to appear on the stage but systems of care centred around population-based prevention were evolving with a lineage that went back to Duncan, Snow, Chadwick, Bentham, and Simon.

The therapeutic era of public health

The Public Health Movement with its emphasis on environmental change lasted until the 1870s and was, in time, eclipsed by a more individualistic approach ushered in by the development of the germ theory of disease and the possibilities offered by immunization and vaccination. As the most pressing environmental problems were brought under control, action to improve the health of the population moved on first to personal preventive medical services, and later to a range of other initiatives including the development of community and school nursing services and school health services. That it was possible to contemplate whole school population measures at all was as a result of the extension to universal education following the 1870 Education Act. This second phase also marked the increasing involvement of the State in medical and social welfare through the provision of hospital and clinic services. As for the arrangements of those involved in the professional delivery of public health services, there was a medical hegemony with a Chief Medical Officer at the national level and local public health leadership provided by Medical Officers of Health. Apart from occasional lecture series such as those provided by Duncan at the Royal Institution or his contemporary Greenhow at St Thomas's in London, formal education was some time in coming. The first course of postgraduate training leading to a diploma in state medicine or public health (DPH) was at Trinity College, Dublin in 1871, to be followed by Cambridge in 1875. These qualifications came under the supervision of the General Medical Council in 1886 and in 1888 it became a requirement that the Medical Officer of Health of any district greater than 50,000 population should hold a diploma in public health. The present situation of a robust multidisciplinary public health workforce was still 100 years off!

The second phase of public health was in turn superseded by the therapeutic era, dating from the 1930s with the advent of insulin and the sulphonamide group of anti-microbial drugs. Until that time there was little of proven efficacy in the therapeutic arsenal. The beginning of this era coincided with the apparent demise of infectious diseases on the one hand and the development of the welfare state in many developed countries on the other. In 1911 in the United Kingdom, Liberal Prime Minister Lloyd George had put in place the building blocks of a National Health Insurance Scheme that would, in due course and after two world wars, culminate in the British National Health

Service dominated by hospital provision. This period came to be characterized by a weakening of departments of public health and a seemingly irreversible shift of power and resources to hospital-based services and particularly those based in teaching hospitals.

Lessons from the pioneers

To quote Sidney Chave once more: 'How can we sum up the life story of this man, the medical officer of health? Conceived by Chadwick, born in Liverpool, he grew up in London and served his apprenticeship there. Thereafter his work took him to every corner of the Kingdom. Wherever dirt and disease were to be found, he was there' (2). So what lessons does 'he' bequeath us? I have identified quite a few:

1. Serendipity favours the prepared mind.
2. The Romans and Greeks got there first. Plagiary is not a crime in public health.
3. The importance of an independent voice, standing up to dogma and vested interests. Advocacy.
4. Data, intelligence, evidence, and annual reports. Shoe leather epidemiology.
5. The power of a local focus, of coalition building, and of organization.
6. Resourcefulness and pragmatism.
7. Humanitarianism and a strong moral tone. A focus on inequalities and enlightened self-interest.
8. Communication and public mobilization.
9. The importance of strong leadership and multidisciplinary teamwork.
10. The necessity for sustainable organizational arrangements.
11. A galvanizing idea, e.g. 'The Sanitary Idea'. Never waste a good crisis. Focus upstream on the determinants. Ride the downward curve of epidemics.
12. The need for education: public, political, professional.

References

1. **Cicero**, *De Legibus*, Book 3, 3, 8, contained in **G. Benham**, *Benham's Book of Quotations: Proverbs and Household Words*. London: Harrap, 1948.
2. **Chave, S. P. W.**, *Recalling the Medical Officer of Health: Writings*, ed. **Michael Warren** and **Huw Francis**. London: King Edwards Hospital Fund for London, 1987.
3. **Chadwick, E.** *Report on the Sanitary Condition of the Labouring Population of Great Britain* (1842), facsimile edition, ed. **M. W. Finn**. Edinburgh: Edinburgh University Press, 1964.

4. **Frazer, W. M.**, *Duncan of Liverpool: An Account of the Work of Dr W. H. Duncan Medical Officer of Health of Liverpool, 1847–63*. London: Hamish Hamilton, 1947.

5. **Finer, S. E.**, *The Life and Times of Sir Edwin Chadwick*. London: Methuen, 1952.

6. **Lewis, R.A.**, *Edwin Chadwick and the Public Health Movement 1832–1854*. London: Longmans, Green and Co, 1952.

Further Reading

Ashton, J., and **J. Ubido**, Healthy cities and the ecological idea. *Journal of the Social History of Medicine*, 4(1), 173–81 (1991).

Marmot, M., *The Health Gap: The Challenge of an Unequal World*. London: Bloomsbury, 2015.

Rosen, G., *A History of Public Health*. (1958), MD Publications, New York. Republished: Baltimore: Johns Hopkins University Press, 1993.

White, B. D., *History of the Corporation of Liverpool, 1835-1914*. Liverpool: Liverpool University Press, 1951.

Whitehead, M., The health divide, in P. Townsend and N. Davidson (Eds), *Inequalities in Health: The Black Report*. London: Penguin Books, 1992.

Wilkinson, R., and **K. Pickett**, *The Spirit Level: Why Equality is Better for Everyone*. New York: Penguin Books, 2009.

Wohl, A. S., *Endangered Lives: Public Health in Victorian Britain*. London: Methuen, 1984.

Chapter 2

Public health at its peak— the interwar years

Following the carnage of the First World War there was a public mood for change that was to be echoed 30 years later, after the Second World War; however, this failed to survive the economic recession of the 1920s and 1930s. The high death rates from the war itself, together with low birth rates, demonstrated that the country could not afford the prevailing infant and maternal mortality, with 1000 babies dying each week. The campaign to reduce infant mortality led with the slogan 'It is more dangerous to be a baby in England than a soldier in France'. The next few years were marked by a battle to extend public health measures which were hindered by what was described by one commentator as 'an ineffectual and parsimonious Local Government Board' (1). A major issue was the departmental division of responsibilities for health and education which was resolved in 1917 by maternity and child welfare services being taken over by the newly formed Department of Health. This left responsibility for the School Medical Service with the Board of Education. Key protagonists in these arguments included the social reformers Sidney and Beatrice Webb, influential Medical Officers of Health George Newman and Arthur Newsholme, and the permanent secretary to the Board of Education, Sir Robert Morant, who held that 'the physical condition of the child lies at the basis of everything educational as well as at the base of the State' (1). He called for the medical inspection of schoolchildren to be expanded to include treatment. The context of these changes included the impact of the Health Insurance Act of 1911, associated with Liberal Prime Minister Lloyd George, with provision for general practitioners to be responsible for the care of working men under the system of panel registration, funded by compulsory health insurance through a partnership of worker, employer, and state, leaving women and children to find what assistance they could through the Poor Law provisions, local government, or voluntary associations.

The ferment of ideas about public health at this time was greatly influenced by Sir George Newman who had become the first Chief Medical Officer in the Ministry of Health and Charles Winslow, the foundation dean of the new School of Public Health at Yale, who clearly shared similar thoughts. For Newman, 'The science and art of medicine is not restricted to the diagnosis and cure of disease in its gross forms ... It is, in fact, the science and art of Health, of how man may live a healthy life at the top of his capacity of body and mind, avoiding or removing external or internal conditions unfavourable to such a standard' (1). Winslow's definition, later to be revived by England's Chief Medical Officer in the 1980s, Sir Donald Acheson, goes into greater detail of what we would now call a whole systems approach:

> Public Health is the science and art of preventing disease, prolonging life and promoting physical health and efficiency through organised community efforts for the sanitation of the environment, the education of individuals in principles of personal hygiene, the organisation of medical and nursing service for the early diagnosis and preventive treatment of disease, and the development of the social machinery which will ensure to every individual in the community a standard of living adequate for the maintenance of health. (2)

This logic paved the way for a programmatic approach to health protection and improvement which was to return in the 1940s with fully fledged plans for a welfare state; and in the 1970s and 1980s when the World Health Organization would describe the elements of a modern health care system grounded in public health. In the meantime Newman's list of principal components of a national policy in preventive medicine seems remarkably contemporary, even if the language is old fashioned and laden with negative connotations as in the case of eugenics:

1. Eugenics and the principles of sound breeding
2. Maternity and the care, protection, and encouragement of the function of motherhood
3. The health and physique of the school child and adolescent
4. Sanitation and an improved personal and domestic environment
5. The prevention and treatment of infectious disease
6. The prevention and treatment of non-infectious disease
7. The education of the people in hygiene
8. Research, inquiry, and investigation; and extension of the boundaries of knowledge.

Although infectious disease is still prominent, and sanitation still mentioned by name, there is a hint here of the beginnings of the forthcoming importance of non-infectious disease and hygiene is clearly prominent.

According to Walter Holland, the Medical Officer of Health (MOH) in the United Kingdom reached (his) peak in 1929. Although the Ministry of Health had been founded in 1917, the next decade had been dominated by the challenge of housing and providing for Prime Minister Lloyd George's 'Homes Fit for Heroes', and progress began to run into the sands of global economic crisis. In 1929 the Poor Law was abolished and its responsibilities, including those for the relief of poverty, passed to local government with workhouse hospitals becoming municipal ones under the direction of the MOH. For Sidney Chave:

> just think of his position now. He was responsible for the traditional environmental services of water supply, sewage disposal, food control and hygiene, for the public health aspects of housing, for the control and prevention of infectious disease, for the maternity and child welfare clinics and their attendant health visitors and midwives; he was responsible for the TB dispensary and the VD clinic; then under his other hat he was in charge of school health, now to all this was added the responsibility for the administration of the local hospital. The MOH was now at the height of his power—this was the peak of his [*sic*] career. (3)

It was the situation that, according to Sidney Chave, would prevail until the advent of the National Health Service.

The hegemony of the Medical Officer of Health may now have been all but complete but it did not mean that there was no rumbling in the ranks of other professionals and members of other emerging professional groups. Duncan's original work in Liverpool had been dependent on good team working involving Newlands and Fresh, engineer and sanitary inspector, but their salary differentials reflected differences in their status within the borough council with clear medical institutional leadership. Mike Eastwood, a former Chief Environmental Health Officer for Manchester, reports from his researches that tensions were to be found, for example, between the Inspector of Nuisances and the Medical Officer of Health. In an editorial in the *Sanitary Inspectors Journal* of January 1896 we find that:

> Whilst we do not counsel insubordination in any respect, we must urge all inspectors to, as far as possible, carry out both the spirit and the letter of the Public Health Acts by preparing and submitting their own reports direct to the Authorities. It is very regrettable to find that in so many cases the Medical Officer of Health obtains the necessary information from the Inspector and dresses it up as his report, when as a matter of fact, the work done by the Inspector he reports upon, he knows little or nothing of, but desires to take credit for ... No doubt it is difficult for Medical Officers of Health to show such a record to justify his existence without such assistance as the Inspectors' reports give him; but it is quite clear that the Acts never intended that the work should be done and reported in this way and we trust that the Inspectors will be strong, and without sacrificing their position, claim the right to prepare and submit their own reports. (3)

Tensions such as these would only grow, and would become part of the story of the demise of the Medical Officer of Health as well as the birth pangs of a new multidisciplinary public health which was still some decades away.

The coming of the welfare state: Straws in the wind

If the foundations of the welfare state can be traced back to the work of social and public health pioneers in the nineteenth century, to the interdepartmental committee on 'physical deterioration' following the Boer War, to Lloyd George in 1911, and to initiatives in the aftermath of the First World War, it was by no means a story of linear, upwards, and onwards progress.

In 1919, Sir Bertrand Dawson, later Lord Dawson of Penn, had been commissioned to chair a council to advise on a comprehensive system of health services. His report concluded that the organization of medicine had become insufficient and was failing to bring medical knowledge within reach of all citizens. He recommended that preventive and curative medicine should be brought together by general practitioners based on a system of doctor's surgeries, primary and secondary health centres, and modern hospitals. His insight into the importance of hospitals being integrated into a whole system remains apposite today: 'Capital expenditure in a hospital differs from capital expenditure in business, in that when a business house grows, it grows in earning capacity, but when a hospital grows, it grows in spending capacity. And therefore almost without exception every hospital in the country is facing increasing difficulty in carrying out its work' (4).

Lord Dawson's proposals for a health service based on health centres fell initially on fertile soil, with bold experiments in some parts of the country. Swindon, which has sometimes inaccurately been described as the birthplace of the National Health Service, was an important reference point. In keeping with the benign paternalistic tradition of other nineteenth-century employers such as the Quaker chocolate makers Rowntree and Cadbury in York and Birmingham, respectively; the textile magnates, Robert Owen in New Lanark and Sir Titus Salt in Shipley; and soap pioneer William Lever in Cheshire, who took a general interest in the wellbeing of their work forces, which extended to housing and recreational provision, the Great Western Railway in Swindon recognized that a healthy workforce was a productive one. Based on a medical fund society and a works doctor in 1847, the companies' facilities had included a swimming pool, Turkish and shower baths (1868), a small cottage hospital in the railway village in 1871, and a works undertaker! Following the Dawson recommendations, a modern hospital with 80 beds and X-ray facilities was planned for 1930 but this along with many other progressive initiatives fell foul of the 1920s depression, the Wall Street Crash of 1929, and the Great Depression which followed it. Times were very hard for millions of working-class families and infrastructure

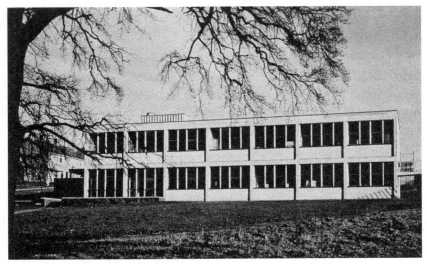

Figure 2.1 Peckham Pioneer Health Centre.
Reproduced courtesy of John Ashton.

spending largely stopped until war clouds gathered once again in Europe and mobilization to fight fascism put everybody back to work.

Two celebrated health centre initiatives which did go ahead were those at Finsbury Park in 1935–8 and Peckham in 1935, both in London (see Figure 2.1).They continue to inspire health system pioneers nearly 100 years later.

Finsbury Health Centre and Peckham Pioneer Health Centre

According to Peter Davey, Finsbury Park Health Centre 'is a monument to social idealism' and was inspired by architect Bertold Lubetkin's belief that 'nothing is too good for ordinary people' (5). When the building was completed in 1938 the area of Finsbury was dominated by slum housing with little in the way of green space and beset with a sickly population. Lubetkin, a Russian Jew who had trained in several European capitals, had seen at first hand some of the utopian architecture to come out of the revolution.

Built to a high, modernist specification, the building captured the progressive ideals of modernism. The building was designed with a commitment to serve a deprived community, to optimize sunlight with a courtyard area and terrace, and included lecture room facilities. It's characterized by an impressive curved facade, 'a smile' Lubetkin once said, sandwiched between what he referred to as 'out stretched arms'—a warm welcome. Reflecting the medical problems of the day, one of its clinics was dedicated to the treatment of tuberculosis. Sadly although the health centre is grade 1 listed, it has not been well maintained over the years.

The Peckham Pioneer Health Centre (Figure 2.1) remains the most ambitious and influential initiative of its kind in the United Kingdom from the 1930s. The initial idea of the Peckham Centre arose from the meeting of two people, Dr G. Scott Williamson and his colleague Dr Innes Pearse, later to be his wife. Williamson was a pathologist who had become fascinated by the lack of susceptibility to disease which accompanies health, and is different from acquired immunity. He sought conditions under which health was to be found and could be encouraged and studied, and this led to the idea of the health centre. On the other hand, Pearse's experience in the early 1920s was in one of the earliest infant welfare clinics in a working-class district, where she gained the conviction that advice on the control of conception should be given in the context of the family as a whole.

The health centre which emerged in 1935 from the ideas and work of these pioneers, together with architect Sir Owen Williams, was and remains a remarkable building. It consists of three large concrete platforms, one above the other, with cantilever supports surrounding a large rectangular central space, occupied by a swimming pool on the first floor. The outer walls and those of the swimming pool were of glass, while the front of the building contained a series of bow windows with sections which could fold back to form open balconies. The building featured partition walls between rooms, allowing flexibility in the use of the floor area.

On the second floor there were private consulting rooms, reception rooms, changing rooms, a small laboratory, and rooms for craftwork and meetings. At one end of the swimming pool was a gymnasium and at the other a theatre which could also be used for badminton. The swimming pool was overlooked on one side by a self-service cafeteria and on the other by a recreation room used for dancing. The ground floor contained a day nursery with room for an infant dormitory.

In planning the new centre it was felt that the population should be essentially healthy and that it should include a cross section by age. It would be for people to come to the centre rather than for the centre to proselytize, and what happened in the centre would be for the members to decide. It would be continuously available in leisure time and its aim was to provide opportunities whenever an opportunity could be taken up—a reflection of the strong belief in Montessori theories of child development.

The scientists themselves were to become one of the groups forming part of the cultural diversity of the centre, and their task was to observe the actions of the individual and the family—and their interactions—as well as carrying out physiological studies of each individual and each family.

The knowledge collected by the scientists was then to be returned to each family for their own use.

The initial equipment consisted of a few books in the library, a billiard table, games for the children, and a piano. The intention was that the family members would acquire and furnish the equipment that they wanted for themselves. The pioneers saw the centre as a building to be furnished with people and with their actions, and they achieved a design which invited social contact. It was to be a comfortable place providing a focus of the sort provided in former times by the village hall and green.

In keeping with the philosophy of the centre as a community resource any family within one mile of the centre could join. This was regarded as 'pram walking distance'. There was to be a family subscription of one shilling per week which brought with it responsibilities and privileges of membership:

- A periodic health overhaul of each individual of a member family.
- The use of the centre and its equipment. This was to be free for all children of school age belonging to a member family, though adults were to pay a small additional sum for each activity.

The community aspect of the centre was underwritten by principles which may well be fundamental to the pursuit of health:

- There was no organizer. It was for the members to organize and choose for themselves how the building would be used. There was an emphasis throughout on self-determination which was symbolized by the self-service cafeteria, a method of organization arrived at by choice rather than expediency.
- Emphasis was on ordinary achievement. Experts were not allowed to dominate any activity by taking it over. This created an atmosphere where everybody felt able to try activities, and not be afraid of failing or being mediocre.

From its opening in 1935 until it was interrupted by the bombing in the Second World War, the Peckham Experiment continued to develop with increasing numbers of family members and a growing sense of identity and loyalty. The building was evacuated at the beginning of the war at the request of the police and was later used as a munitions factory. Twenty-nine young families with 50 children under 5 years of age went to live at a farm in Bromley which had been acquired by the Peckham Centre and which was wanted by its members to provide fresh food and milk. However, the country experiment apparently failed for financial reasons after about a year.

The facilities at Peckham Health Centre

For its time the Peckham Health Centre included an impressive range of facilities and services;

1. Welfare and educational

   Antenatal clinic; postnatal clinic; birth control clinic; infant welfare clinic, care of the toddler; nursery school; immunization service; schoolchildren's medical examinations; vocational guidance; sex instruction for adolescents; girls' and boys' clubs; youth centres; sports clubs and recreation clubs of all sorts; keep-fit and gymnastic classes; adult cultural education; music, debates, drama, any event desired by members; citizens advice bureau; holiday organizations; outings and expeditions; the bar; billiards; dancing; social gatherings.

2. Therapeutic

   Marriage advice bureau; mothers clinic; child guidance; poor man's lawyer; social worker; hospital follow-up overhaul; rehabilitation clinic.

In 1945, as a result principally of the demand by former members of the centre, the building was reopened, and of the 875 families who were members before the war, 550 families immediately rejoined. Over the next 3 years, however, the financial support available to maintain the building proved inadequate and in 1951 the pioneers were compelled to sell the building to the local authority, initially for use as an adult education centre.

Ironically, support for the centre had not been forthcoming from the National Health Service when it was established in 1948. Apparently the ethic was not compatible with the ascendant values of the therapeutic era and the rise to domination of hospital-based care. However, the seeds of Peckham took root elsewhere and have continued to influence the work of progressive thinkers and innovators in the intervening years until today.

The fall and rise of public health

The therapeutic era of public health can be dated from the 1930s, with the advent of insulin and the sulphonamide group of drugs and later of penicillin. Until that time there was little of proven efficacy in the therapeutic arsenal. The discovery and artificial production of insulin transformed the management of type 1 diabetes and has saved millions of lives worldwide. The definitive breakthrough in identifying the hormone was by Banting and Best in the early 1920s in Canada and it led quickly to the availability of the first therapeutically usable supplies derived from animal sources. The first sulphonamide, Prontosil, was discovered by the chemist Josef Klarer in Germany in 1932 and by the late

1930s was making a significant contribution to the treatment of serious infections, saving the life of the son of United States President Franklin D. Roosevelt and playing a central role in the treatment of Second World War wound infections before the availability of penicillin. Penicillin itself was discovered by Alexander Fleming at St Mary's hospital in London as early as 1928 but it was not until 1944 that it went into mass production, just in time for the Allied invasion of Normandy. Professor Jerry Morris, one of the founders of post-war public health at the London School of Hygiene and Tropical Medicine, was to describe how, as a young army medical officer in India and Burma, he was the first person to use penicillin in the field and was disciplined for disobeying orders by driving 50 miles over difficult terrain to obtain a supply from an American army unit for a soldier who was very sick but who survived.

The beginnings of modern pharmacy and pharmaceuticals coincided with the apparent demise of infectious diseases and a subsequent weakening of departments of public health with a shift of power and resources to hospital-based services. General practice was a particular casualty of the immediate post-war period. Later this was to contribute to the commonly held view that all improvements in health were a result of scientific medicine and that improvements in health were as a result of a National Health Service and its clinical interventions. It would not be until the 1970s that this point of view would be challenged by Birmingham professor of social medicine Thomas McKeown.

Newman's comprehensive view of a public health system had been gaining traction since the 1920s and in 1941 historian Sigerist noted that any national health programme ought to include:

1. Free education including health education

2. The best possible working and living conditions

3. The best possible means of rest and recreation

4. A system of health institutions and medical personnel available to all responsible for the population's health, ready and able to advise and help them in the maintenance of health and in its restoration when prevention broke down

5. Centres of medical training and research.

Perhaps William Morris's 1884 definition of health best captures the enduring sentiment underpinning the efforts of many of those striving to protect and improve public health:

> At least I know this, that if a person is overworked in any degree they cannot enjoy the sort of health I am speaking of; nor if they are continually chained to one dull round of mechanical work, with no hope at the other end of it; nor if they live in continual sordid anxiety for their livelihood; nor if they are ill-housed; nor if they are deprived

of all enjoyment of the natural beauty of the world; nor if they have no amusement to quicken the flow of their spirits from time to time; all these things, which touch more or less on their bodily condition, are born of the claim I make to live in good health. (6)

The economic recession of the 1920s and 1930s and the misery it brought to millions in poverty, followed by the horrors of global war and the immediacy of the German blitzkrieg of British cities with thousands of civilians killed, were beginning to impact on policy thinking. In November 1942 Lord William Beveridge reported to the British Government in a plan for 'Social Insurance and Allied Services' in a document which represented an emerging consensus of what would be needed once the war was over. Huge queues formed outside the Government Stationery Office in London and the report was sold out by lunchtime. Beveridge's plan was put forward as part of an attack on the 'five giant evils':

the physical Want with which it is directly concerned, upon Disease which often causes Want and brings many other troubles in its train, upon Ignorance which no democracy can afford among its citizens, upon Squalor which arises mainly through the haphazard distribution of industry and population and upon Idleness which destroys wealth and corrupts people whether they are well fed or not, when they are idle. (7)

The Beveridge report struck a chord with a population worn down by 20 years of economic adversity and world war, one in which a remarkable resilience and sense of social solidarity was to be the legacy. In 1945, the British people rejected the war-time leader Winston Churchill in favour of a radical socialist programme headed up by Clement Attlee with a Welshman, Aneurin Bevan, as Minister of Health and Housing. This would see through the ambitious aim of creating a National Health Service for the whole population. It is fascinating now to see how clear the connection still was between the environmental focus on housing and the clinical services to be provided by hospitals and family doctors. That Churchill had been taken by surprise by the strength of feeling of the British people coming out of the sacrifices of war has been attributed in part by the solidarity created in the battlefield by all social classes rubbing along together for a common end—the defeat of fascism; observers have also pointed to the political education and awareness raising in the field brought about by classes run by the Workers Education Association.

The National Health Service which was inaugurated in 1948, at a time when the country was technically bankrupt, was intended as one major plank of post-war reconstruction, reflected in other countries through the creation of their own public health and related services and collectively through the creation of the United Nations (UN), the World Health Organization, and the other UN agencies, to address the root causes of social instability, conflict, and war. When it was implemented, the NHS had a tripartite structure, consisting of, firstly, the existing regional civil defence-based war-time networks of poor law and municipal and university hospitals; secondly, the family doctors, opticians, pharmacists, dentists, and other community health services; and thirdly, the accumulated community health services including maternal and child health clinics and venereal disease clinics together with the extensive range of other activities of local authority-based public health services under the direction of the Medical Officer of Health.

This tripartite structure brought with it a set of tensions arising from conflicting governance arrangements and the compromises which Bevan had found necessary to deliver the National Health Service. In part these tensions were at the root of the dysfunctional recurring intervention by politicians in the ensuing decades, unable to resist the temptation to embark on periodic structural reorganizations. For many years commentators appeared to have lost sight of this profoundly important concept of an integrated tripartite set of arrangements. Perhaps, most importantly, it was lost sight of in the wholesale structural change affecting local government in 1974, when the post of Medical Officer of Health disappeared and the public health functions were redistributed and fragmented. In recent times there has been an effort to retrieve that integration with the publication of the Five Year Forward View by the Department of Health in 2014, the development of New Care Models emphasizing integration, partnership, and prevention, and the movement of responsibility for public health back into local government from the health services themselves, where it had landed in 1974.

Underpinning the decline in public health during the immediate post-war years was the advent of science-based medicine, in particular as manifested by the fruits of the pharmaceutical industry. This industry was to experience phenomenal growth over the next few decades with investors flocking to put their money in what came to be seen as 'blue chip' investments. In the meantime tuberculosis, that 'captain of the men of death', continued its retreat along with a long list of childhood infections such as diphtheria, whooping cough, measles, mumps, and polio, as vaccines became available and could be delivered to whole cohorts of children through delivery systems based on the National Health Service. Even epidemic pneumonia began to wane as antibiotics became available and these same antibiotics were there to deal with the complications of infection. An indication of the shift that was taking place comes from the fate of the Peckham Pioneer Health Centre, a place- and population-based initiative with a focus on prevention and primary care. In the immediate aftermath of war and with hospitals in the ascendancy, it failed to secure funding and passed out of use as a health facility.

Meanwhile, recruitment to public health began to suffer as hospital careers beckoned and the Empire of the Medical Officer of Health began to ebb away. Paddy Donaldson, one of the last Medical Officers of Health who worked in Yorkshire and the North East of England in the 1950s and 1960s, has left us a glimpse of the end days of the golden years when his role could include the hospital, the port, the schools and child health clinics, and the triumph of victory over childhood epidemics together with the mopping up of the last cases of pulmonary tuberculosis.

Infectious diseases appeared to be on the run and the future held out the promise of 'a pill for every ill'. New priorities began to emerge as Europe emerged from the shadow of mass unemployment and war and standards of living rose. At the same time the new National Health Service was beginning to uncover questions of need, demand, and supply as a commitment to population coverage exposed the challenge of resourcing 'an equal service, free at the time of use' and of equal quality. Perhaps those pioneers of a National Health Service held a rather naive view that once universal care was available and a backlog of disease brought under control, progressively less resources would be needed for a healthier population. We had yet to fully understand the layers of onion that can be a population's health need and demand and the long-term consequences of creating expectations of professional care for even minor problems with its consequent negative impact on self-care and the lay health care system. Straws in the wind of the extent of unmet need in those early days were the crises brought about by patients coming forwards for spectacles and for dental treatment who had long been invisible, suffering in silence, but who now began to put resource questions high on the political agenda.

Changing emphasis and fashion were not the only threats to the position of the medical officer of health as he (*sic*) moved into the 1960s and 1970s. The huge hierarchical departments remembered by Mike Eastwood in Manchester and Liverpool were also coming under threat from internal tensions generated by the aspirations of emergent professional groups. Those colleagues in environmental health, social work, and nursing, who had long played second fiddle to the public health doctor, were becoming restless with desires for their own professional space and autonomous practice. In retrospect the challenge can be seen as that of finding multi- and interprofessional ways forward. In effect, the 1974 Local Government reforms which swept away the Medical Officer of Health, following on from the hiving off of social work in 1970, and which led to separate directorates and spheres of influence of brother and sister professionals, created unfortunate silos, with often dysfunctional relationships. The tripartite arrangements of 1948 were on their way out and Humpty Dumpty had fallen off the wall. It was to be 40 years before a serious attempt would be made to reintegrate the essential components of a whole public health system. A great deal of water would flow under the bridge with multiple structural reorganizations. One thing that wouldn't go away would be the underlying philosophy of a National Health Service for the whole population with an enduring emphasis on inequalities in health.

References

1. **Holland, Walter W.,** and **Susie Stewart,** *The Rock Carling Fellowship 1997 Public Health: The Vision and The Challenge,* pp. 34 and 38. The Nuffield Trust, 1997.
2. **Winslow, Charles Edward A.,** *The Untilled Fields of Public Health.* Science, 1920.
3. **Warren, Michael,** and **Huw Francis** (Eds), *Recalling the Medical Officer of Health: Writings by Sidney Chave.* King Edwards Hospital Fund for London, 1987.
4. **Dawson. B.,** Interim report on the future provision of medicine and allied services 1920. London: Ministry of Health, 1920.
5. **Davey, Peter,** Lubetkin's Finsbury Health Centre—the ideal that time forgot. *Architectural Review.* B D Magazine—Healthcare, March 2009. Available from https://www.bdonline.co.uk/lubetkins-finsbury-health-centre-the-ideal-that-time-forgot/3135725.article
6. **McKeown, T.,** *The Role of Medicine: Dream, Mirage or Nemesis.* London: Nuffield Provincial Hospitals Trust, 1976.
7. **Beveridge, Sir W.** *Social Insurance and Allied Services.* Conditions 6404, 6405. London: HMSO, 1942.

Further Reading

Donaldson, R. J. *Off the Cuff. Reminiscences of My Half Century in Public Health.* Richmond, Surrey, UK: Murray Print, 2000.

NHS England, Five Year Forward View. 2015.

Pearse, Innes, and **Lucy H. Crocker,** *The Peckham Experiment: A Study of the Living Structure of Society.* London: George Allen and Unwin, 1947.

Sigerist, H., *Medicine and Human Welfare.* Oxford: Oxford University Press, 1941.

Part II

The three pillars of public health

Chapter 3

Improving health in Mersey

In the early 1980s the National Health Service in England had a similar number of regional health authorities to when the NHS had been established in 1948. The regional tier was a strategic one, which had an important role in reconciling competing demands for investment in hospitals and estate, for manpower, contingency planning, ambulance services, blood transfusion, and many other functions. At that time the typical regional authority contained architect and legal departments, human resources, and a staff complement running into many hundreds. There would be a medical department led by a regional medical officer with close links to the local medical school and local hospital doctors, and a nursing department with a regional nurse who held a hierarchical position between the chief nurse in the Department of Health in London and the thousands of nurses employed in the region. Each local borough within the region would have a local health authority with operational links to the local hospitals and their medical and nursing committees. Since 1974, the responsibility for public health had moved from local government to the NHS, with community medicine consultants and teams based in local health authorities and the regional level. The Regional Medical Officer was construed as having a clinical orientation, facing the hospital and medical world and being 'the doctor's doctor', but with a minimal public health orientation.

In 1988, as a result of weaknesses in the new arrangements that were manifested by a failure to deal effectively with outbreaks of infectious disease, Sir Donald Acheson carried out a review of the public health function, which led to its strengthening through the recruitment of a new national cohort of trainees, the creation of joint posts for communicable disease control between health and local authorities, the abolition of the job title of 'community physician' and its replacement by 'director of public health' and the reintroduction of the requirement that directors of public health should produce independent annual reports. For some of us the opportunity was missed to embrace a multidisciplinary workforce, something for which we had to wait almost 15 years. It is against this somewhat messy background that a new generation of public health workers was trying to create a movement for a new public health and beginning to use the language of 'health promotion'.

Taking up my new post in Liverpool at the beginning of 1983, I was to be working from a public health base in the university medical school combining teaching commitments with the medical students with the development of my research interests. In addition, as was commonplace at the time, I had an honorary consultant contract with the Mersey Regional Health Authority covering a region of 2.4 million people, centred on the City of Liverpool and the two counties of Merseyside and Cheshire in the North West of England. Usually medical school academics held such contracts which gave them access to patients and to clinical responsibilities in addition to their teaching and research; in the case of public health there was a general confusion about what exactly should be the clinical responsibilities accompanying an honorary contract and it was common for these to be interpreted very sparingly, often amounting to not much more than weekly attendance at the regional medical officer's staff meeting.

In contrast, I had been much influenced by the recognition that historically there had been two parallel models of academic public health in operation. The first model was one in which the old-time Medical Officers of Health had been simultaneously the local professor with teaching commitments, usually with quite superficial research interests apart from the occasional publication of a case study of some practical, albeit important, public health intervention; an example of this might be the publication in the *Lancet* in 1959 of a description by Liverpool Medical Officer of Health (MOH), Dr Andrew Semple, of an incident of Anthrax at Liverpool docks. With the second model, in some universities a different tradition had grown up, more deeply rooted in research and often involving large-scale epidemiological studies and trials, divorced from the everyday practice of public health.

With the demise of local authority public health departments this latter model was in the ascendancy, which to my mind was to the detriment of both parties and to public health. I was much taken by the view of London School of Hygiene and Tropical Medicine's Professor Geoffrey Rose that public health practitioners should have 'clean minds and dirty hands', that the work of practitioners should be rooted in up-to-date evidence, and that if practicable they should be research active; whilst the work of public health academics should be rooted in the messy day-to-day work of public health policy and practice. Whilst working as a senior lecturer at the London School of Hygiene and Tropical Medicine, with an honorary contract with one of the London health regions, I had endeavoured to make the practical role a meaningful one, but with limited success. Expectations were low and resources not forthcoming. I had managed to convene a coronary prevention team, and assembled a team of prominent members from academia and service but its activities never progressed beyond the 'talking shop' stage. Nevertheless, this experience would not be wasted in Liverpool.

Getting a face on the New Public Health

The job description for my new post at Liverpool included that of health promotion with the Regional Health Authority. This new term was just beginning to catch on and the use of the term enabled the authority to look as if it was keeping up with current trends. In reality, the incumbent Regional Medical Officer was an old school 'doctor's doctor' type with little feeling for the modern agenda. The university honorary contract holders were invited to a weekly meeting at which he smoked his pipe as we watched the lunchtime ferry leave Liverpool Pier Head for the Isle of Man. The only rule of the meeting was that there should be no agenda, and very little of consequence was ever discussed. On one occasion a new senior lecturer from the Liverpool School of Tropical Medicine turned up for the meeting unannounced and uninvited; within days the regular attendees received a letter from the Regional Medical Officer pointing out that this person who had turned up was unknown, uninvited, and unwelcome and please could we discourage him from returning. Dr David Nabarro went on to have a highly distinguished career in global health both with the World Health Organization and the United Nations. It was not an encouraging start. However, things were about to get better with the appointment of a new chairman of the Regional Health Authority who believed in getting things done, and a new chief executive who would go on to become the chief executive of the NHS in London. In the meantime, it was a question of digging deep for resourcefulness; fortunately there were some clues to be had.

As a young medical student in Newcastle in the late 1960s, I was fortunate to share a flat in Jesmond which had for years been occupied by medical students. The owner, a retired naval officer living on the ground floor, Basil Houghton was a wonderful old man; although suffering from advanced Parkinson's disease he never let this get in the way of his work as a volunteer fundraiser for the London Missionary Society. From early in the morning as we left to go into lectures, he would be bashing away on an old typewriter with one finger, sending off letters seeking donations for the cause. One summer morning, on my way out I passed him sitting on a rug by the paling fence at the front of the Holly Avenue garden with a can of paint in one hand and a brush in the other. 'The important thing', he said, 'is to get a face on it.' That evening as I returned from a full day he was just finishing off.

When Edwin Chadwick wrote to William Henry Duncan enquiring as to his establishment, Duncan replied to the effect that 'the following is my entire establishment, your servant William Henry Duncan' (1), whilst one of my mentors in Newcastle, psychoanalyst and gastroenterologist Bill Brough, would often use the analogy from deep sea diving of 'buddy breathers', in which two divers going down together have the security that if one had a problem with their oxygen line they could both share the other. In my career I have been privileged and fortunate to have had not only a remarkable stream of mentors but also a succession of buddy breathers. Even the most challenged environment has assets and even the most disadvantaged community has leadership waiting to be recognized and supported. These timeless lessons are at the heart of modern public health. In January 1983, arriving back in Liverpool with a mandate to promote the health of 2.4 million people, I needed to get a face on it.

My debt to three men

In the public health work that I would become immersed in for the next 40 years there were three men whom I would honour for giving me a leg up and a start. Firstly, there is Sidney Chave, already mentioned a number of times, who not only revealed to me the nature of my vocation, but also introduced me to William Henry Duncan, an iconic figure in public health of whom I was ignorant up until then and was largely unknown in his own city until the 1980s, and unacknowledged nationally. Through his teaching Sidney demonstrated the importance of communication, populism, and creativity in making public health visible, tangible, and real. There is a story I like to tell my students of two men on a train in Africa. One of the men goes to the window and begins to throw powder out of it. The second man asks what he is doing. 'Throwing out powder to keep the elephants away', says the first. 'But there are none', says his friend. 'There you are', retorts the first, 'it works'. An important task of public health is to make prevention visible.

Public health movements, not precious, arcane public health practices, were what Sidney Chave was talking about, even when exploring the role of one man in Duncan. Storytelling and biography were an instinctive part of his repertoire. Sidney's three photographs of schoolchildren from the East End of London, taken at 25-year intervals, told a powerful story of poverty, social conditions, growth, development, health, and wellbeing. The first photograph, taken around 1900 at the time of the Boer War, shows a group of ragged-trousered boys, looking short and stunted, some of them with no shoes, many of them looking tired and drawn with the clinical signs of chronic upper respiratory infection. As a local priest was to remark to me later of the boys he worked with in a disadvantaged part of Liverpool, 'the light has gone out of their eyes by the age of 12'. By the time of the second photograph, the immediate impression was of taller, fitter, better turned-out lads; even in the aftermath of the First World War, with the economy faltering, and the recession looming, nutrition and living conditions had improved. And by 1950, two years into the welfare state with the benefits of the NHS and following a sustained period of egalitarian food rationing during the war, the public health dividend of these measures was beginning to become apparent.

These lessons of storytelling, of communication, and of engaging the public in its public health history were not lost on me. Sidney's inspired idea to have two London pubs renamed and themed to tell the stories of public health pioneers John Snow and Jeremy Bentham paved the way for us to do the same thing for Dr Duncan in Liverpool and in so doing begin a process of taking a great story and inspiration out of the library, onto the streets and into public consciousness (see Figure 3.1).

Sidney's message about Duncan as 'the local boy made good' spoke to me personally about the legitimacy of working locally and making a contribution close to the community as opposed to being seduced by the glittering prizes of servicing national institutions and elites.

A second important influence was Dr Tom Hobday, a pragmatic conservative of the old school, who gave me a most precious gift when I arrived back in Liverpool—the gift of his time, his wisdom, his knowledge, and his networks. We were poles apart politically but shared a passion for the city, its people, and its public health. Tom had combined the roles of Conservative politician on the city council, where he was chairman of the Health Committee, with being a colonel in the Territorial Army with responsibility for health emergency planning throughout the era of the Cold War with the Soviet Union; on his wall in the Regional Health Authority were to be found the secret maps of emergency rest centres and other defensive installations in the event of a nuclear war. In addition he had held down the position of senior lecturer in public health at the Liverpool Medical School, a position which I was about to inherit from him. Tom took me for a long lunch at the Liverpool Athenaeum where he shared decades of insight and guidance, saving me months if not years of legwork and challenge. In public health we are united in a noble mission where even those we disagree with can be allies.

The third major input came from Dr David Player, one time Chief Executive of the Health Education Council in London. When he heard that I was leaving London to return to the North West, David charged me with developing a programme in Liverpool to tackle the twin problems of teenage pregnancy and

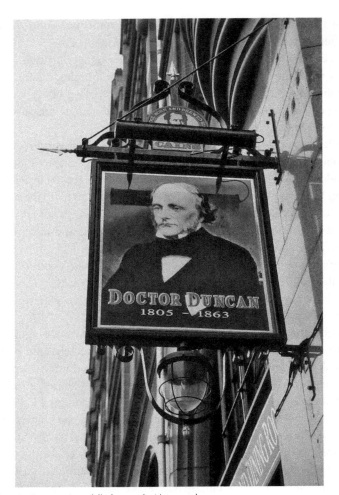

Figure 3.1 Dr Duncan's public house in Liverpool.
Reproduced courtesy of John Ashton.

sexual health and his finance officer Don Freeman found the funds to get it started; Don Freeman was one of those rare finance officers who asks what it is you are trying to do and then goes looking for the resources to make it possible. David Player was also somebody who led by example and put the health of the public before self-interest. In 1986 I was with him during the landmark Health Promotion conference in Ottawa, Canada, when he was summoned home by the Minister of Health to be sacked from his post; his crime, to compare publicly the marketing of low tar cigarettes as a healthier product with jumping from the twentieth rather than the thirtieth floor of a skyscraper!

Intelligence is the basis of public health action

In using a regional health authority and a university department of public health as a platform from which to launch the New Public Health, the World Health Organization's strategy of Health for All by the Year 2000 was taken as the starting point. Beginning from a low base of public health activity in 1983, the next ten years were to present some remarkable challenges but together we were able to demonstrate effective interventions that encompassed the promotion of healthy lifestyles, coming to terms with the current phenomenon of high teenage pregnancy rates, heading off the terrible threat posed by the advent of HIV/AIDS in a population afflicted by high rates of heroin injection, and dealing with a range of external threats to health including other new infections and environmental disasters. By the time I left the university to take up the full-time position of Regional Director of Public Health and Regional Medical Officer, not only had we reinstated Liverpool's leading position in public health and its role as a training centre, but had laid the foundations of a resilient public health system for the North West region.

The ecology of the Mersey region

In 1983, the Mersey Health Region was the smallest and most compact of 14 National Health Service regions with a 2.4 million population centred on the City of Liverpool, and the two counties of Merseyside and Cheshire to the north and south of the great River Mersey, respectively. Within a matter of years and through a crazy series of structural reorganizations of the National Health Service it would be absorbed into a new North West Region with an administrative headquarters in Manchester, a territory bounded by the Scottish Borders and the Pennine hills, and a population approaching 8 million, second in size only to London. The region encompassed a cross-section of the nation in the variety of its geographical and physical appearance, in its social structures and activities, and in the health of the people it contained and supported; 1 in 20 of the population of England and Wales lived within the Mersey Region, which showed marked contrasts in the conditions of life between industrial, urban, and rural areas.

To an extent the City of Liverpool and its surrounding districts dominated the region. From its modest beginnings as a fishing village on the River Mersey, Liverpool's history has reflected and anticipated that of much of the rest of the region and of the country. The city's commercial growth dates from the late seventeenth century, although most of its fabric dates from the nineteenth century and later. The Port of Liverpool was founded on the slave trade and the notorious triple passage of the slave ships between Liverpool and West Africa where manufactured goods were exchanged for human cargo, which was then transported to the Americas where people were sold on as slaves, before the ships returned to Liverpool with the lucrative bounty of cotton, tobacco, and rum. It became the first port of the British Empire with more millionaires than London and a truly cosmopolitan population mix that included descendants of the Great Irish Famine refugees, Welsh builders who roofed the tens of thousands of terraced houses with Welsh slate, and the oldest African and Chinese populations in Europe. These, along with others from maritime countries, found their way to Liverpool aboard ships, and settled among the local people. However, economic decline followed the Second World War with the end of the British Empire, the demise of the transatlantic passenger trade, and, more recently, the migration of company head offices to the south east of the country to be nearer to Brussels and the European Union. We were left with the decaying remnants of the obsolete docklands, an infrastructure of inner city deprivation and health inequalities, appalling unemployment rates, and newly created social problems appearing in overspill housing estates where social relations had often fragmented.

Eating an elephant (you must start somewhere)

The notion that if you are about to eat an elephant it is necessary to start somewhere, but that knowing the shape of the task in hand is a useful notion in public health. As Duncan and Snow showed, clear simple data transformed into intelligence is the basis of effective public health action. The lessons to be drawn from Sidney Chave's writings are no less important, not least the need for bold leadership, resourcefulness, pragmatism, serendipity, organization, and communication. John McKnight, the father of Asset-Based Community Development and a great storyteller, is fond of reminding us that 'you don't go to the store until you have seen what you have in your backyard'. There are resources to be found, both human and environmental, in all communities, however disadvantaged.

Most public health problems are quite obvious and indeed are staring us in the face: poor housing and homelessness, unemployment and hazardous work, poverty and inadequate nutrition, pollution of the air, water and food, the brutalization of children growing up under deprived conditions, lack of recreational facilities, and poor access to basic health care and safe maternity services. Simple ethnography and statistics are usually adequate to define what is happening—in essence shoe-leather epidemiology. The first steps to creating the New Public Health in the Mersey region involved bringing together a team and developing a strategy based on a community diagnosis.

Establishing the first multidisciplinary regional health promotion team

Establishing the first multidisciplinary health promotion team in the country was greatly assisted by a change of personnel at the top of the organization. The new chairman was Sir Donald Wilson, a larger-than-life 'Marmite' figure whom you either loved or couldn't stand. Sir Donald was a political appointment during the administration of Margaret Thatcher as Prime Minister; a dairy farmer in the county of Cheshire, both Sir Donald and his wife, Lady Edna, were prominent members of the county Conservative Party. The stories of his idiosyncratic approach to management were legion but one thing clear to me was his passion for the National Health Service, his commitment to it and his unwillingness to let anybody harm it, on his watch, in his region. This was not a doe-eyed passion but rather one forged in a traditional and paternalistic conservatism and from the cut and thrust of the business world. From the outset I enjoyed his support and I like to think that he recognized in me a shared passion to do the best for the people of Mersey and, later, the North West.

We were fortunate, too, in the appointment of the new Chief Executive, Duncan (later Sir Duncan) Nichol, and when he was called to head up the NHS in London, his successor Geoff Scaife. All these men brought to the task a thirst for innovation and creative solutions, which was exactly what we needed to get started. They subscribed to a prominent idea from one of the business school texts of the time, namely that if you look at the top performing companies that remain in the top league year after year, one of the common features is that they have within them a maverick group enjoying the protection of the top team that can innovate, take risks, and approach problem solving and intervention from left field. We were doubly blessed. That Sir Donald Wilson could straddle the style of NHS paternalist and innovator whilst keeping the politicians in London happy was to prove a particular boon.

When Duncan and Snow were facing the challenge of cholera in the 1840s and 1850s, life was hard but in some ways simpler. The society of the day was highly ordered and paternalistic, and ordinary people did not expect to take part in decision-making; rather, they knew their place. The MOH had considerable institutional authority but the range of possible interventions was usually limited. Even when public health expanded into personal health services there was no strong consumer lobby and the power of the town hall was considerable until at least the post-war years.

By 1983 the situation was much changed. Contemporary health problems were almost inevitably multifactorial and the prevailing social ethic largely libertarian. Unlike the opportunity to provide safe drinking water which was available to the Victorians, there were few straightforward measures that could bring immediate results. Action on tobacco, seat belts, or fluoride might present themselves as such examples, but when examined closely could be more problematic; for an initiative to be successful the climate of opinion needed to be such that the public regarded it as helpful and desirable and a measure which they wished to go along with and defend. The widespread flouting of the prohibition of cannabis was perhaps a good example of this and we have seen in the intervening years how the decriminalization agenda has been edging forward under public pressure; on the other hand, the public supported increased restrictions on the use of tobacco products when this impacted on the freedom to breathe fresh air. The battle for compulsory seat belt use took many years to be won and required a concerted approach for mass education backed up eventually by legislation; the fluoridation of water supplies as a measure for improving population dental health, whilst fully evidence based, became bogged down for years through the orchestrated opposition of opponents.

The achievement of lasting change in the factors affecting health and disease nowadays involves taking the public with you. The World Health Organization has long advocated 'making the healthy choices the easy choices' and for several decades governments have shied away from legislative solutions for fear of being accused of representing 'The Nanny State'. This reluctance to use all the tools at its disposal has not served public health well, for example in relation to the disastrous effects on child health and obesity levels and the rise in the prevalence of Type Two diabetes from the failure to legislate on junk food and sugary drinks. There are limits to the effectiveness of an approach based on 'nudge'!

If by the early 1980s the style necessary for modern prevention had come to be seen as participatory, Peter Draper and his colleagues in London had made a strong case for multidisciplinary health promotion teams that could work in harmony with each other and with the public. In their terms there could be no more 'medical heroes' in the mould of the MOH. Such teams needed to be an independent resource to the community and capable of taking on vested interests without fear of losing their jobs, a condition of service recognized as necessary so many years before in Liverpool.

The first step was to set up a multidisciplinary regional health promotion team within the Regional Health Authority based on six principles which had been identified as catalysts for a New Public Health movement:

1. Activity on health promotion and disease prevention should be carried out at the most decentralized level that is compatible with effective action.
2. There should be a multidisciplinary team approach.

3. Participation by the community should be an overriding principle.

4. Health promotion teams should have security of employment and freedom of action.

5. A strategic plan for the promotion of health should be produced at the regional level that is informed by the priorities and objectives decided at the periphery.

6. Health promotion teams should produce annual reports based on the development of appropriate indicators that can be used to assess progress and revise objectives.

The most important initial function of this team was to obtain access to the range of resources that existed within the Health Authority and to open up internal channels of communication to influence the priorities of the Authority. It subsequently evolved to include stakeholders from outside the health services as it began to develop a broader role of influencing the whole system impacting on health. A significant moment came with the securing of the salary for the country's first Regional Health Promotion Officer (Howard Seymour), an experienced Health Education Officer and social entrepreneur who quickly opened up access to the health authority's planning process and budgets and developed wide-ranging links with both statutory and non-statutory bodies. This marked the beginning of the first phase of development, agenda setting, to be followed by consciousness raising of public health issues at a community level together with the development of models of good practice which illustrated the putting into practice of the philosophy of 'Health for All'.

At this time public health had been in the shadows of clinical medicine for several decades. It had become divorced from the main institutions, including those of local government, which have influence over many of the determinants of health. Further, there was a major issue in that those who had an important part to play in improving and protecting health were often not aware of their own significance. It is said that Mark Twain was writing prose for twenty years before he knew that that was what he was doing because he was ignorant of the meaning of 'prose'. In the same way, many of those in civic society, voluntary organizations, and local government had assumed that health services were responsible for health when in fact their focus was almost exclusively on treating disease. In this they had been denying the true health agencies the recognition and support for their contributions, whilst failing to deliver on their own important contribution to public health. This needed to be addressed and would be a long journey.

As those in the new field of Health Promotion began to grow in confidence, some made the mistake of claiming that the New Public Health should be entirely non-clinical. There were two potential errors in thinking as we felt our way forward; the first error was to continue in the belief that public health was still owned by medicine, whilst the second was to think it could do without it. Thirty years on we have a rich mixture of public health trainees, team members, and leadership roles including those of directors of public health who are drawn from a wide range of backgrounds; these include education, environmental and social science, the humanities, and community organization and development, as well as the biological sciences and clinical disciplines.

In the meantime, the task in hand was to share with many people across the Mersey region that indeed they were and could be writing and practicing health prose. The starting point was to be the country's first regional public health report, *Health in Mersey*.

Health in Mersey—A Review

The reference point for a systematic approach to public health was a community diagnosis, *Health in Mersey—A Review*, which was published in 1984. This was the first such public health report for any English region and marked the beginning of a recognition of the regional level as being an appropriate one for public health strategy, innovation, and facilitation. It was intended to provide a strategic framework for the region of 2.4 million people, with its many local health authorities and their accountability to their communities.

The power of timely and relevant information is at the heart of public health, and is its bedrock, as the work of the early pioneers so clearly shows. Epidemiology, statistics, and social enquiry underpin the stories that can lead to effective policy and action. Yet too often the apocryphal Finagles Law applies in that the information we have is not the information we need and the information we need is not available. By the 1980s there was increasing interest in the re-energizing of local public health reports but the climate of the times was emphasizing financial and accountancy data at the expense of the clinical and of health outcomes. Whereas in the 1850s John Simon had placed great store by having the vital statistics for the previous week on his desk every Tuesday morning, at health authority top team and board meetings it was commonplace for the finance officer to have pole position on agendas and to come armed with abundant printouts of the latest financial returns. In contrast, discussions of public health were often an afterthought with little investment in capacity with which to generate the relevant intelligence.

The production of a community diagnosis

One central part of preparing the groundwork for a public health strategy was rec-ognized to be agenda-setting for key opinion formers and decision makers within the region. Despite the ten years of discussion about prevention since the publica-tion of the Lalonde Report in Canada in 1974, and a series of prevention-orientated reports which had followed it, confusion persisted at a local level about what health authorities and other statutory and voluntary bodies should actually be doing.

Moreover, there seemed to be a considerable ignorance of the wider context, including that of the World Health Organization strategy of Health for All by the Year 2000. If there was to be any prospect of developing a concerted, multi-sectoral approach to health promotion based on the extended concept of pri-mary health care espoused by the WHO, it would be necessary to produce a document which placed local health data firmly in a local context, and drew clearly on the WHO strategy. The target for this document was to be local poli-ticians, members of health authorities, local authorities, and health watchdogs and other community groups and charities with a health interest, together with health staff of all kinds within the region. Lalonde's notion of the need to influence the entire 'health field' in which health determinants and influences play out was implicit in the scope of the work which needed to be done for whole systems change. The intelligence provided needed to reflect this.

In the absence of dedicated public health resources within the Regional Health Authority it was necessary to win over and mobilize resources from across the organization in support of what was proposed, an asset-based approach rem-iniscent of the challenge faced by the Health of Towns Association members in the 1840s. The compilation of the report required the committed support of the statistics section of the Health Authority with a willingness to work closely with the author, who had an overview of what was needed. This overview was not initially shared by the statistical staff. It also required the identification of es-sential non-health service databases such as those relating to education, social services, and the police, and the collation of such data, which was not routinely used by the Health Authority (see Table 3.1). The assistance of a part-time re-search worker was provided by the regional health authority for this purpose.

Additional analyses were carried out by the regional health authority statis-tics section to refine the data for presentation, to enable district comparisons to be made, and to construct novel indices such as the Standardised Years of Life Lost Ratio prior to age 75. At this time it was normal to take 65 years as the nor-mative age for mortality analyses, but the remarkable increases in general life expectancy were just emerging.

Table 3.1 Types and sources of data used in the production of *Health in Mersey*

Type of data	Source (*n*) number of organizations
Census data related to living and working conditions. Fertility and mortality statistics	Office of Populations Censuses and Surveys (OPCS)/ Regional health authority/county councils (2)
Hospital morbidity data (hospital activity analysis)	Regional health authority
Family doctor preventive medical services and other family doctor data	Family Practitioner Committees (5)
Health authority preventive medical services. Community health manpower and resources.	District health authorities (10)
Special educational needs data	Local education authorities (5)
Road traffic deaths, narcotics and other offences	Merseyside and Cheshire County Constabularies (2)
Chronic sickness and disability	Local social services (5)
Consumer interests	Community health councils (11)

Format of the report

The outcome of the work described was the production of a 90-page report written in plain English, which could be easily understood by the informed lay reader. The assistance of an interested local graphic artist working pro bono was obtained in presenting visual material in an attractive way. The report was intended to present a historical and ecological account of health within the region, and to highlight the major causes of premature death and disability and the priorities for health promotion at each stage of the lifecycle (see Box 3.1).

For each of these topic areas a section was written synthesizing the necessary action for a concentrated approach to health promotion. The resources and expertise available for health promotion within the region were reviewed, and the facilitating and hindering factors identified where this was possible.

Handling the report and consciousness raising

The report *Health in Mersey—A Review* was initially produced for the first Mersey Health Promotion conference held in the town of Warrington, in the centre of the region, in April 1984. This conference formed a briefing for 550 key opinion formers and decision-takers from around the region. The

Box 3.1 Contents of *Health in Mersey*

Chapter 1 The nature of the health field

Chapter 2 Defining the problem—The determinants of health

Chapter 3 Health in Mersey—The ecology of the region

Chapter 4 The population of Mersey health region

Chapter 5 The causes of death and ill-health

Chapter 6 Prevention or cure—The development of a strategy for health promotion

Chapter 7 Health for all by the year 2000

Chapter 8 Twelve priorities for Mersey

Chapter 9 A strategy for action including information and research needs

From a review of the state of health within the region and the discussion of health strategy in other countries, twelve priority topics for health promotion in Mersey emerged (see Box 3.2).

Box 3.2 Priorities for *Health in Mersey*

1. Planned parenthood
2. Control of sexually transmitted disease
3. Antenatal care including genetic screening
4. Improved child health and increased immunization uptake
5. The prevention of death and disability from accidents and environmental causes
6. Improved dental health
7. Some specific aspects of lifestyle related to premature death (including diet, exercise, stress, tobacco, alcohol, and drugs)
8. The effective control of high blood pressure
9. Early detection of cancer
10. Reduction of disability in the elderly
11. Dignity and comfort at the time of death
12. A healthy mind in a healthy body—positive health especially as it relates to a health strategy for young people

intention was to acquaint them with best practice from around the country and to set an agenda for action based on the findings of the report, which would cross the boundaries of discipline and agency. Participants were to leave the conference with a copy of the report and the stimulus of the ideas to which they had been exposed. When they returned to their own authority or organization they would begin to question what they could and should be doing about the 12 priority topics and how best to support any initiatives to take them forward. This was the beginning of the process of consciousness raising across the wider community of the agenda for action and the scope of the new public health.

The conference and the report itself were extensively covered by the local and regional mass media. Subsequently, the in-house resources of the regional health authority print room were deployed to produce over 10,000 copies of the report, with distribution extending widely to include the members of the many organizations represented at the conference who were in a position to act. The report, with its 12 priorities for action, became the basis of a chapter in the Regional Health Authority Strategic Plan; it was incorporated into district health authority planning priorities, and was so mainstreamed. Finally, and of importance for the reorientation of professional practice for the future, it became standard teaching material for medical, nursing, and health visitor students in the region.

The strength of response to the publication of the yellow report across the agencies that had been engaged paved the way for innovative action aimed at addressing the 12 priorities. The immediate follow-through focused on the parallel tracks of developing a review process which could be used to monitor the implementation of health promotion strategies at the district level together with appropriate indicators and targets to underpin them.

The review process

The review process was intended to be a non-threatening means of engaging with district partners based on the responses to a questionnaire about the 12 priorities. In all some 200 questions were asked, defining what activities were being pursued in each district in relation to these topics. It was felt important only to ask questions to which at least some of the districts could respond affirmatively, making the exercise a positive one. Replies from the 10 districts were collated and laid out in a way which made comparison easy. These were made available for discussion within the districts, and provided the basis for the district review meetings. Agreement was then negotiated between the districts and Regional Health Authority on specific initiatives to be taken over the following 12 months.

Information and intelligence for the New Public Health

The WHO Health for All strategy had devoted much consideration to the information requirements necessary to support global and national action. WHO had recommended that 'before 1990, member states should have information systems capable of supporting their national strategies for Health for All' (2). Such information systems, it was held, should provide support for planning, monitoring, and evaluation of health development and services, assessment of progress towards Health for All, and dissemination of relevant scientific information; steps should be taken to make health information easily accessible to the public.

The production of the *Health in Mersey* report was an example of an attempt both to set an agenda for health promotion in the region and to make health information readily accessible to the public. However, during the course of producing the report many of the deficiencies in the current information system became apparent. In particular it was clear that much routinely collected data of relevance was not at that time being made use of because it was collected by non-health agencies. In addition, the lack of useful local as opposed to regional or national data, especially in relation to lifestyle and preventable risk, highlighted the need for new approaches.

As a direct result of this a working party was convened to examine information needs under the chairmanship of the Regional Chief Statistician. The terms of reference of the working group were to examine the 12 priority topics from the point of view of developing an information strategy around them. The approach adopted was essentially that which had been used nationally to produce an information strategy for the National Health Service itself. This consisted mainly of identifying the minimum data sets required to provide information under the following headings:

1. Demand (as a proxy for need)
2. Inputs (resources available)
3. Outputs (workload, population coverage, process, and organizational aspects)
4. Outcomes (state of health)
5. Environment (including social, economic, and psychological influences)

The structure of information needs

Five categories of data were identified:

1. Health service data—Data which was readily available but needed to be organized and presented in a useful way.

2. Related organization data—Data covering a wide range of organizations which is often readily available once arrangements have been made for it to be supplied.

3. Special survey data—This forms a significant part of the data needed for health promotion and may be resource intensive. Typically, it needs to describe the local environments that influence and shape health behaviour and choice. It is needed to supplement routine statistics and enable the monitoring of progress on health goals. Survey techniques of the 'dipstick' or cross-sectional market research type, allowing periodic assessment of small area based populations are likely to be the most productive.

4. Analytically derived data—Typically, these relate to small area statistics for economic and social variables. Fundamental data are often available such as those based on the national census or national surveys, but they may need to be analysed in relation to a specific variable or specific level of disaggregation.

5. Soft descriptive data—A complete understanding of each priority topic at a community level requires qualitative data employing the rich perspectives of anthropology, social, and behavioural science.

The outcome of the deliberations of the working party was to identify a small number of specific indicators in relation to each of the 12 priorities. For each of these indicators its currently available status was identified either as:

◆ Available now

◆ Analysis required

◆ Development work or special survey required.

Three criteria were applied for individual indicators:

1. That they should stimulate change by the nature of their political visibility and punch, through being sensitive to change in the short term and being comparable between places.

2. That they should be simple to collect, use, and understand, be directly available now or available in a reasonable time at a reasonable cost.

3. That they should be related to health promotion.

This approach was subsequently adopted in a WHO workshop on Healthy Cities held in Barcelona, leading to the so-called 'Barcelona Criteria' in 1989.

The selection of the indicators and targets was not intended as a final list but as a starting point to facilitate comparison between districts and to encourage debate. The emphasis of the proposed data was on small area comparisons and the reduction of health inequalities. Part of the development work that was needed for each priority was to enable an accurate description of the context or 'health field', in which each topic was but an epiphenomenon; that that context should take account of relevant legislation or implicit or explicit public policy and such social, cultural, and organizational factors as impinged on people's ability to influence their health status. The context statement for each priority was best seen in relation to the development of Health Impact Statements capturing the impact of formal or informal health policy and in which the impact of policy in non-medical sectors was made explicit. Between them, context and health impact statements could provide the bridge of intelligence, monitoring, and research for multi-sectoral action.

In the ensuing years the necessity to develop compatible data bases between local and health authorities has continued to be a struggle, not least because of constant structural reorganizations and the loss of corporate memory.

Suggested indicators and targets for the 12 Mersey priorities

For each of the 12 health promotion priorities a succinct position statement was developed based around a framework which included indicators, a statement of context, a proposed target, and an underlying rationale. This can be illustrated by reference to three of the priorities: planned parenthood (see Box 3.3), the prevention of death and disability from accidents and environmental causes (see Box 3.4), and some specific aspects of lifestyle related to premature death (see Box 3.5).

The Mersey Strategic Framework

One of the challenges for those working in public health is the sheer breadth of its remit. All aspects of living and working conditions, the ways in which we interact with our biology and environment and the institutional and organizational arrangements that we create, impact on public health. The very origins of local government are rooted in the challenges that people face for protection of their health at the local level. The need for a whole systems approach can seem overwhelming and the transformational ideas contained in the WHO policy and strategy documents utopian. When *Health in Mersey* was published one response from traditional officers within the Regional

Box 3.3 Priority 1: Planned parenthood

Proposed indicators (available now):

♦ 15- to 19-year-old conception rates

♦ Proportion of conceptions resulting in a live or stillbirth for age groups 15–19, 20–24, 25–34, and 35–44.

Context statement: Availability and characteristics of relationships education (including birth control), accessibility and acceptability of contraceptive services to all social groups.

Proposed target:

♦ That by the year 2000 the conception rate for 15–19 year olds in all districts should be 14/1000 or lower.

Rationale: This level of teenage pregnancy had already been achieved in the Netherlands with a broadly similar pattern of teenage sexual activity. As an indicator this was a good summary of the outcome of relationships between education and the accessibility and acceptability of birth control services to all social groups.

Box 3.4 Priority 5: Prevention of death and disability from accidents and environmental causes

Indicators (available now):

♦ Number of days NO_x or SO_2 exceeded WHO guidelines

♦ Home ownership by tenure and type

♦ Proportion of households suffering from overcrowding

In addition a number of indicators on accidents in the home, on the road, at work, or sustained during recreation were available and a small amount of additional analysis and data on water pollution could be made available with the cooperation of the water companies. Other than this there was a range of development work needed, especially in relation to qualitative indicators of the environment.

Context statements: The existence of fully staffed departments of environmental health in local authorities with adequate mechanisms for public consultation and for liaison with health and other relevant agencies.

Box 3.4 Priority 5: Prevention of death and disability from accidents and environmental causes *(continued)*

Proposed targets:

1. That by the year 2000 deaths from accidents of all kinds should have been reduced by at least 25 per cent through an intensified effort to reduce traffic, home, occupational, and recreational accidents.

2. That by the year 1990 all districts should have fully staffed departments of environmental health in local authorities in accordance with nationally derived staffing norms. These departments should have adequate mechanisms for public consultation and for liaison with health and other relevant agencies.

3. That by the year 1990 a clear picture of chemical pollution risks to the domestic water supply should have been established and a plan drawn up to eliminate them; that measures would have been developed to assess consumer satisfaction with the taste of drinking water and regular consumer surveys begun to be carried out. That by the year 1995 chemical pollution of the water supply should have ceased to occur and public satisfaction with the taste of drinking water should exceed 95 per cent of the adult population.

4. That by the year 1995 there should be no days in the year on which NO_x or SO_2 levels exceeded WHO guidelines.

5. That by the year 1990 the increasing trend of episodes of food poisoning should have been reversed and a system of training courses in the nutritional aspects of food established for food handlers in retail outlets and cafes in both the public and private sectors.

6. That by the year 1995 the major known health risks associated with the disposal of hazardous wastes should have been eliminated and bathing beaches within the region should all have reached European Union standards.

7. That by the year 2000 the proportion of households suffering from overcrowding in the most disadvantaged local government ward should be the same as that in the most advantaged ward.

8. That by the year 1995 all employers will have made adequate arrangements to monitor work-related risks and have agreed a prevention strategy with their workforce and with the surrounding population.

Box 3.4 Priority 5: Prevention of death and disability from accidents and environmental causes *(continued)*

Rationale: The environmental area is a central one in public health. It was felt that at that time there was a need to move away from traditional structural indicators which tended to be readily available towards process and functional indicators of environmental quality which needed to be developed, particularly through market research techniques. One contemporary example of the use of traditional indicators was to be found in the Swedish city of Gothenburg where data lineage between the police, hospitals, city engineering, and town planning departments had led to traffic management changes with resultant reductions in loss of life and serious injury.

Box 3.5 Some specific aspects of lifestyle related to premature death

Indicators (available now):

- Unemployment rates
- Proportion of children receiving free school meals
- Proportion of school leavers continuing into higher education of various types
- Household car ownership
- Premature years of life lost and hospital bed days used by cause

Context statement: Control over resources related to lifestyle through time, e.g. accessibility to low-cost, high-quality food for people on low income and the possession of knowledge and skills to take advantage of it.

Proposed targets:

1. By the year 2000 mortality from diseases of the circulatory system in people under 65 years of age should be reduced by at least 15 per cent and the death rates in the most disadvantaged wards should be the same as those in the most advantaged.

2. By the year 2000 the current rise in male suicide and attempted suicide rates should be reversed and the decline in female rates should be sustained.

3. By 1990 all districts should have systematic programmes of health education to enhance the knowledge, motivations, and skills of people

Box 3.5 Some specific aspects of lifestyle related to premature death
(continued)

to acquire and maintain health and each school should have at least one teacher designated as having responsibility to coordinate health education.

4. By 1995 in all districts there should be established trends in positive health behaviour such as balanced nutrition, non-smoking, appropriate physical activity, and good stress management. Indicators of these trends should be available at local government ward level and the differences between the most advantaged and disadvantaged wards in health knowledge and behaviour and biological status should be narrowing.

5. By 1995 in all districts there should be established downward trends in health-damaging behaviour such as overuse of alcohol and pharmaceuticals, use of illicit drugs and dangerous chemical substances, dangerous driving, and violent social behaviour. Indicators of these trends should be available at ward level and the differences between the most advantaged and disadvantaged wards in health knowledge and behaviour and biological status should be narrowing. By the year 2000 the proportion of the population living in the most disadvantaged ward and engaged in satisfying work should be the same as that of people living in the most advantaged ward.

Rationale: The lifestyles area is a central one to public health and health promotion. It was felt in the 1980s that there was a need to move away from traditional indicators of mortality and morbidity which tended to be readily available towards more functional process indicators of the quality of life and of its determinants. Very often such indicators were more of a horizontal nature in that a cross-cutting factor such as 'locus of control' or 'sense of coherence' might have an impact on a range of behaviours related to such matters as self-esteem. Narrowly medical or biological and disease indicators can serve to reinforce a silo mentality in prevention and lead to an inefficient deployment of resources with multiple interventions focused on individual disease outcomes. This way of thinking might have seemed novel as the New Public Health unfolded, but in retrospect what was the Victorian emphasis on environmental action but a series of horizontal measures such as slum improvement and safe water supplies that impacted on many different diseases and conditions?

Health Authority was that 12 priorities was far too many when the contemporary wisdom of business and health service management schools was to focus on three.

In my heart I have always believed that a full and comprehensive picture is needed if we are not to become victim to threats to health coming in from the left of field. We need this if we are to be not only systematic about protecting and improving health but also able to seize the moment to progress on particular issues when the opportunity presents itself. A considered response to the assertion that priorities should be limited to three is to ask how many of the biblical Old Testament Ten Commandments are optional?

Putting health intelligence on a firm footing—The Liverpool Public Health Observatory

Using data transformed into intelligence, and marketing it widely to set the New Public Health agenda, was to become a leitmotif for modern public health practice. It echoed the work of the early Medical Officers of Health which was grounded in 'registration, notification and advice' (3); the evidence base of timely, hard-hitting reports and populism was the guiding theme. As the local health authorities on Merseyside increasingly realized the value of this kind of intelligence against a background of increasing frustration with more traditional academic outputs, whose timeliness was often in question, they were persuaded to support the UK's first Public Health Observatory in the Liverpool Medical School which was established in 1990. This first Health Observatory was based on the local authority observatories to be found in other European countries.

At the time of establishing the Liverpool Observatory the problem of conventional funding of research and intelligence from the universities was seen as being the tendency to take the funding and disappear for several years, only to come back with the answer when the question had changed. Questions needing to be answered in days, weeks, or months rather than months and years did not fit in with the universities' research timetable and did not seem to be valued. At the same time public agencies and non-governmental bodies needed robust and reliable intelligence including 'shoe-leather epidemiology' to shape policy options and decisions. The alternative of free floating consultants often proved shallow, disconnected, and ephemeral. Was there not scope for a win–win situation by packaging the work that needed to be done within an academic environment but with contractual safeguards so that the needs of all stakeholders could be met?

Box 3.6 Liverpool Public Health Observatory: Examples of topics covered after 1990

- Planned parenthood
- Family planning, abortion, fertility
- Coronary heart disease and stroke
- Drug misuse and drug misuse services
- Alcohol abuse, needs assessment, and service review
- Deafness
- Asthma and environmental pollution
- Tuberculosis and poverty
- Cystic fibrosis and deprivation
- Health impact assessment of the Merseyside integrated transport strategy.

This idea of developing health intelligence in observatories had resonance in other initiatives which were emerging at the time. In the United States Kerr-White, dean at Johns Hopkins School of Public Health had suggested that each medical school should have a centre for health intelligence linked to the dean's office which could influence the education and training of students by matching curriculum to local population health needs. In Europe the World Health Organization was to establish a European Observatory together with a network of academic centres to promote the development of evidence-based health policy; and in 1999 a new government in the United Kingdom picked up the idea of public health observatories from Liverpool, encouraged by Chief Medical Officer Sir Liam Donaldson. In her health strategy 'Our Healthier Nation' Public Health Minister Dame Tessa Jowell proposed a regional network 'in order to strengthen the availability and use of information about health at the local level we will ensure that there is a Public Health Observatory in each ... region of the country' (3). As I moved from the University of Liverpool in 1992 to become Regional Director of Public Health it became timely to review the function of the original observatory in the light of recent developments. The upshot of this was to establish a second observatory for the whole region based at Liverpool John Moore's University. This new observatory was much more grounded in a commitment to multidisciplinary public health and would go on to play an essential role in supporting local Directors of Public Health in their general

Box 3.6 Liverpool Public Health Observatory: Examples of topics covered after 1990 *(continued)*

need for intelligence, whilst becoming a national and international centre of expertise in work on behavioural aspects of public health including alcohol, drugs, HIV/AIDS, sexually acquired infection, and violence as a public health issue. Meanwhile, the original observatory established went on to establish its reputation for health impact analysis.

The harvest that I was able to reap in my work for the North West was rich, with a comprehensive range of powerful reports on a wide range of topical matters that enabled us to make a real impact. A novel example was the production of a health calendar which made explicit the chronology of health issues around the year, and a report on the weather as a public health forecasting tool.

Substantive areas of work which built on the reputation which had been acquired through the publication of policy relevant research into behavioural aspects of public health included that on criminal justice, violence, and alcohol.

◆ The canon of work on criminal justice created a map of overlapping issues including drug use, alcohol, violence (domestic, youth, sexual), abuse, and neglect especially of the very young and of older people, the sex and illegal tobacco trades, together with the trade in other health-harming products, road traffic issues, and health and safety.

◆ The work on violence stemmed from the publication of the World Health Organization's Report on Violence and Health in 2002 and had a significant influence on Public Health Directors in England who would later take on a leadership role in violence prevention and with the WHO publication of international guidance on the primary prevention of violence.

◆ An extensive body of work on alcohol led to a much higher prioritization of the issue nationally than had until then been the case, and often provided data which advocates, such as former President of the Royal college of Physicians Sir Ian Gilmore, were able to put to good use. There had been national guidelines for safer alcohol consumption but these had often been ignored and seen as intangible. The North West Public Health Observatory was able to pin down the empirical evidence for alcohol harms, developing and producing annual local alcohol profiles for England which set out the health, criminal, and economic damage caused by poorly regulated alcohol markets in each local authority area. What followed was an intense period of national and local policy activity where politicians tried to come to terms with the clear harms caused

> **Box 3.6 Liverpool Public Health Observatory: Examples of topics covered after 1990** *(continued)*
>
> by alcohol without damaging the cash cow that alcohol had been for the Treasury for hundreds of years. This saw the UK government re-examine licensing, revisit drinking guidelines, and look again at what part alcohol should play in the lives of children.
>
> As advocates for public health and lobbyists for the industry made their respective cases we saw a minimum unit price for alcohol accepted, first for national policy followed by a near immediate U-turn as the industry lobbyists pulled the various political levers at their disposal. Once the new English public health agency, Public Health England, had been established the regional public health observatories' functions were largely centralized and emasculated. As a result they lost the precious and influential identities that they had developed, becoming part of a bureaucratic national level structure. As so often in public health it often seems to be a case of two steps forward and one step back.

The Liverpool Observatory had as its mission 'to generate and evaluate the application of public health intelligence

1. By anticipating and responding to clients' public health intelligence needs

2. By supporting development of the public health and related organizations

3. By acting as a focus for maximizing the cross-fertilization of experience and skills between academic and service public health to maintain methodological rigour'.

The notion of an 'observatory' was taken to convey standing back from phenomena and events and providing description, analysis, and forecasting of patterns, inter-relationships, processes, and outcomes. By these means it was intended to play a part in healing the schism between academic and service public health. Examples of the many reports produced in the early years of the observatory are contained in Box 3.6.

References

1. Chave, S. P. W., *Recalling the Medical Officer of Health: Writings*, ed. **Michael Warren** and **Huw Francis**. King Edwards Hospital Fund for London. London: WHO Health for All Strategy, 1987.

2. **WHO Health for All**. Available at: https://www.who.int/dg/priorities/health-for-all/en/

3. **Jowell, Dame Tessa**, *Saving Lives: Our Healthier Nation*. Available at: https://www.gov.uk/government/publications/saving-lives-our-healthier-nation

Chapter 4

Promoting and improving health

In the early days of health education the focus was very much on behaviour change. This would later be seen as a narrow and individualistic approach, certainly when compared with the Lalonde whole systems notion of 'the health field' and the ideas about empowerment which were to be promoted in the Ottawa Charter. The emphasis was very much on 'knowledge, attitudes, and practice', a model based on rational control rather than on more recent concepts such as those of 'sense of coherence' or 'locus of control'. The movement for a New Public Health harked back to Richard Titmuss's, of the London School of Economics, emphasis on 'control over resources through time', later recast by the World Health Organization (WHO) as 'making the healthy choices the easy choices'. Relevant too for the evolution of the new thinking had been the framing of three types of health education encompassing, firstly, the traditional approach emphasizing knowledge of biology and behaviour; secondly, consumer information about how to make the most of services; and thirdly, the more contentious and challenging idea of supporting citizens who were fully armed to fight for good health and challenge anti-health forces.

The technical briefing of opinion formers and decision makers is now seen as necessary for a health promotion strategy to succeed, but not of itself sufficient. A parallel process of consciousness raising on a large scale is needed, leading to more effective individual and collective actions to improve health, together with the incorporation of health promotion ideas into the political process from the ground up.

The ensuing logic is that by mobilizing the public through increased understanding focused on the wider determinants of health and their inequalities, not only will individuals become their own health experts but also health citizens. The collective effect of such a phenomenon can be a major improvement in public health as a result of individual healthy choices, supported by increasingly responsive and healthy public policies at a local and national level. Until the 1980s the tendency had been to see consciousness raising as being about campaigns in the mass media aimed at individual behaviour change, an approach which is vulnerable to the charge of victim blaming. The tension between this and a more structural effort directed at the policy determinants of ill-health and inequalities through the use of health advocacy would characterize the next three decades. The charge of the 'nanny state' would become a rallying cry of health free-marketeers as they recycled ideas of social marketing, and later of 'nudging' people into good health behaviour rather than accepting that the primary purpose of government is to protect its citizens from hostile outside forces including such agents as the processed food and soft drinks manufacturers. What was clear was that mass media campaigns in isolation had little chance of achieving long-term effects, and that influencing the entire field in which health choices were shaped was necessary for real progress; this was something that remains well understood by the cigarette industry with its approach to penetrating everyday life with its messages and its insidious normalization of health-damaging behaviour. Increasingly we have seen these cynical approaches adopted by the sugar and soft drinks industry.

Consciousness raising: The example of the Health Promotion Fair at the Liverpool International Garden Festival, 1984

The International Garden Festival, held in Liverpool from April to October 1984, offered a unique opportunity to bring health-related information to a mass audience as part of the new health promotion strategy. The underlying philosophy was one which regarded the large festival site as a whole 'field' or setting, in which positive health influences and messages could be insinuated into the entire visitor experience.

Health was made a major theme throughout the festival with educational material being featured in a number of sites, including the area containing allotments and other horticultural gardens. The festival grounds occupied a dramatic location along the banks of the River Mersey, much of it being contaminated land. The idea of a garden festival had come from Conservative politician Michael Heseltine, who was appointed Minister for Merseyside, by Prime Minister Thatcher in the aftermath of the 1981 riots in the city. Heseltine had a passionate commitment to the regeneration of the northern cities which he recognized as having been the source of the United Kingdom's wealth during the days of Empire; a keen gardener, he had been influenced by the experience of other European countries in using garden festivals to regenerate run-down urban areas.

In the case of the Liverpool Festival the term 'health fair' was used to denote the range of activities rather than a single static base, the objective being to promote active, experiential learning. Activities included static displays, providing information on a range of health matters; dynamic displays, consisting of health-orientated activities such as aerobic dancing, yoga, meditation, and sports; and public participation, involving physical fitness testing and interactive lifestyle assessment. Of the 3.3 million people who attended the International Garden Festival, 250,000 were estimated to have visited the static part of the fair, and most of them made use of one of the first computerized lifestyle assessments producing a personal printout with lifestyle advice; 11,000 actually took a fitness test.

Computerized lifestyle assessment

Twelve computers offered a range of self-operated programmes which included a dental health game, an actuarial assessment of longevity, and an interactive lifestyle analysis. The areas included in the programme were diet, smoking, weight, stress, alcohol intake, and heart disease risk.

Fitness testing

The 56 health promotion assistants who were drawn from the large number of long-term unemployed to be found on Merseyside in the early 1980s were taken on as part of a government-funded job creation programme. Each received training during a two-week induction period which consisted of:

- Education on major health problems and the relationships to lifestyle;
- Instruction in fitness testing and the interpretation of results;
- Instruction in the use of computer facilities; and
- Advice on communication and presentation to the public.

The venue was constantly manned by a rota of staff; the fitness tests used included tests of stamina and grip, flexibility, and body fat.

Twelve months after the initial interview a sample of 234 people who had completed a research questionnaire at the time of their initial contact were sent a further questionnaire to complete themselves. With a response rate of 67 per cent the major finding was that there appeared to have been actual changes in behaviour in the three main topics of the health fair, i.e. diet, smoking, and exercise (24 per cent had an improved diet, 20 per cent were taking more exercise, and 6 per cent were smoking less or had stopped).

An important aspect of health promotion which this programme illustrated was the value of initiatives which combined a whole systems, 'health field' approach, mass coverage, and individual counselling, without compromising quality. This was possible by using a combination of semi-skilled workers and high technology computers—'Hi-tech and Hi-touch'!

Part of the covert health promotion agenda was to provide a positive work experience for the 56 long-term unemployed young people. The staff had the opportunity to be part of a friendly, task-orientated work group, with a great deal of public contact and potential job satisfaction. In addition, they acquired health knowledge for themselves and, indirectly, for their families.

The importance of an emphasis on personal development became self-evident during what turned out to be a remarkable initiative. The success of the Garden Festival Health Fair can be judged from its subsequent continuing development as a mobile phenomenon using five double-decker buses at the end of the summer which continued for several years.

Other aspects of consciousness raising

Taking public health off the shelves of academia and into the streets was an emerging theme of what came to be known as the New Public Health in the 1980s. Sidney Chave had shown the way in London with his imaginative theming of the John Snow and Jeremy Bentham public houses; but this was just a hint of what was needed. Later the John Snow Society at the London School of Hygiene and Tropical Medicine would follow up with an annual 'Pump Handle' lecture commemorating Snow's celebrated intervention in Soho. In Liverpool the transformation of Dr Duncan's pub in Liverpool into a public health theme pub, the commemoration of Duncan's family house, and the establishment of an annual Duncan lecture in the medical school marked the point at which the name of William Henry Duncan was taken out of obscurity and used to rebrand public health for a new age.

The First Duncan Lecture entitled 'Duncan of Liverpool—and some lessons for today' was given appropriately by Sidney Chave. Concluding his inspirational call to action Chave referred to William Beveridge's five giants and concluded that in 1983 Liverpool 'we do not have to look far to find them still. They remain a continuing challenge to all those who are concerned with the well-being of this city and this country … Can we lift our eyes from our desks to meet it? I think we can—I think we should'. And of the future public health practitioners to come, his rallying cry was that 'Would some scribe write of him then, as he once wrote of Duncan; "He is not only a reality; he is a power in the commonwealth" ' (1).

That lecture series continues over 30 years later, having counted among its alumni some of the most prominent figures of the New Public Health.

Populism and public health

A populist approach to consciousness-raising for public health can take many forms, and overlaps with the important work of advocacy. It also links to the idea of an asset-based approach to health. All communities, however challenged, have human and environmental assets which can be mobilized for the protection and improvement of health. In the case of urban areas these include not only community activists but a plethora of environments ranging from schools, libraries, art galleries, and sports facilities to commercial malls, city parks, and other open spaces.

As our work evolved, extensive and regular pro-active exposure in all types of media and at all levels became the order of the day, reaching out and engaging with the population in all the settings of everyday life. Street-level recognition of the work and priorities of public health is essential to the success of its mission. Early examples of taking a visible position on current issues included the withdrawal of health promotion support from a street festival as a protest against the sponsorship of the event by a tobacco manufacturer and a public protest at the choice of Merseyside for test-marketing tobacco chewing pouches.

Pro-active interventions such as these were still unusual at that time but became much more common in later years. It is debatable whether today things have progressed since the return of public health to local government, with constraints being placed on the public actions of local government officers. Issues such as the investment of pension funds in the tobacco industry and the compliant attitude of many towards the continuing activities of the tobacco and sugar industries with new products can be seen as a litmus test of the independence of action of public health teams.

Also at this time involvement with Liverpool Football Club was negotiated at no cost with posters portraying the Championship squad as a no-smoking team; public controversy was generated over the tardiness of milk and dairy distributors in the region in responding to consumer demand for low fat products; and extensive collaboration was developed with the local commercial radio station which included regular prime time health discussion slots, and the transmission of a gold medal-winning special programme on smoking.

Looking back on this work 30 years later, it is gratifying to be able to report on the extent to which such initiatives have become mainstream. It is hard to imagine how unusual it was elsewhere, apart from other isolated examples such as the groundbreaking work by Trevor Hancock and his colleagues in Toronto. When it came to the third strand of strategic action for the New Public Health, that of developing systematic models of good practice, we were able to draw on the emerging experiences from elsewhere.

Developing models of good practice

Innovation in large organizations and whole systems is not easy, and often just when it seems that progress is being made the opposition begins. One of my first meetings after returning to Liverpool was with a local government chief officer who explained the reality to me. 'You have to realize' he said, with the demeanour of experience, 'that when you come out with all these wonderful ideas, they will tell you it won't work'. 'Why not?' you might respond, 'it works in (… Holland, Sweden, Canada …)'. 'Yes, but it won't work here, here is different', followed by a long exposition of the history, the politics, and the myriad of arguments against change. But if you are determined you have to start somewhere, to find the 'buddy breathers' and 'make a face on the job'. What is important is to make both the elephants and the future tangible through the use of stories but also through the realities of demonstration.

According to the diffusion theory of innovation, diffusion takes place through the appropriate social system and individuals, groups, or organizations decide to accept (or reject) the innovation. It can help if there is a good crisis and the innovation can be sold as the solution. As more members of the system adopt the innovation an S-shaped curve is produced, the rate of adoption affecting the steepness of the curve. Stocking described the limitations to this model when applied to the British National Health Service, with examples of changing patient waking times, preventing rickets in Asians, and introducing day surgery. This was in the days before desperate and abortive efforts were made to achieve transformational change through the use of the private market. There are no easy answers, winning hearts and minds is as important as providing sound evidence and data, and there is no substitute for credible, trusted, and authentic leadership.

Institutional inertia is the enemy of innovation and transformation. Successful firms have devices to enable them to continue to innovate after their original product champions have gone or subsided into complacency. One way to break the cycle of inertia, which seems to particularly afflict large bureaucracies, is to have visible models of good practice.

The Karelia Project—A totemic initiative

The systematic, whole population approach, exemplified by the North Karelia Project has already been referred to in Chapter 2. This represented one of the first large-scale modern public health interventions addressing the post-war epidemic of non-communicable disease affecting developing countries. When I visited Finland in the early 1980s on behalf of Professor Jerry Morris to present the recently published 'Black Report' on inequalities in health in England to the Boards of Health in Stockholm and Helsinki, I took the opportunity to visit this project, which was already beginning to attract international attention based on its early positive results. Its leader, Pekka Puska, had used succinct epidemiology from a WHO international study of heart disease to galvanize community action and pressure the Finnish Government into supporting action to do something about the appalling heart disease statistics that had been demonstrated for Finnish men.

The approach adopted by the project not only linked academic epidemiological research findings to policy and community levels of action, but paved the way for public engagement and the new ideas about the reorientation of medical care towards primary care, public health, and prevention and away from a fixation on hospitals. It tackled these challenges by using a small project team to work with existing health service staff and encourage them to work in a different way; this centred on a partnership not only with statutory agencies but with ordinary citizens in their community associations, and with different-sized businesses, including, for example, encouraging butchers to proffer low fat products for sale. At the national level fiscal policies were adopted to make it cheaper to move away from full fat dairy products; some of the first legislative tobacco control measures were adopted in the world; and a systematic approach was taken with the use of mass media for public health education. Regular population-level surveys of nutritional and other relevant behaviours were conducted, detailed studies were carried out on changes in dietary salt intake, and it was all backed up by community case registers of hypertension and heart disease run by family doctors. At the same time a major national initiative was taken to re-engineer capital and workforce investment away from hospitals towards a health care system rooted in primary care. This is something that many countries are still struggling with in the face of entrenched political, public, and professional resistance. Forty years on there has been a dramatic reduction in the level of deaths from heart disease in Finland, as the lessons learned in Karelia have been rolled out across the country.

Of particular interest is that the comprehensive methods developed in Karelia were influential outside of the immediate focus on cardiovascular and other non-communicable disease. In particular the whole systems approach was picked up in adjacent Sweden where it was adopted with important results to address the recent phenomenon of rising teenage pregnancy rates. These followed the discovery of the contraceptive pill and the sexual revolution of the 1960s.

HART—The Health and Recreation Team

The Health Fair at the International Garden Festival provided the platform and the impetus for a range of new initiatives to influence the health field. These included the health promotion buses, the various Duncan initiatives to reclaim the branding of Liverpool's first Medical Officer of Health for the New Public Health, and opportunistic and media activities. Over time they would lead to an extensive range of 'settings'-based work including healthy cities, schools, hospitals, prisons, workplaces, stadia, and night clubs.

The Health and Recreation Team was an initial attempt to take some of the learning from the 1930s Peckham Experiment in London together with the emerging ideas from Finland and use them in a contemporary context. The kind of comprehensive, social, educational, and health centre run on cooperative lines which was pioneered in Peckham is difficult to replicate today, although there are increasing examples of multipurpose community 'hubs' being developed, based on schools, churches, community centres, and even pubs. In Finland the very concept of a health centre is not confined to one building but can include a network of, usually clinical, facilities and frequently beds which can be used for closer to home medical care. This raises the possibility of a 'networked health centre', a functional rather than a physical concept. It should be possible to enter any of these public institutions and readily find the services in the others which are most appropriate to particular needs.

The HART project, funded by the Sports Council nationally, was initially based in one health centre and employed a community development worker. The ambition was to develop networks that related especially to sport and exercise. Extensive, active links were developed between a number of health and community centres together with local government and non-governmental organizations across Liverpool. HART was able to give a considerable boost to the local implementation of the National 'Look After Yourself' programme, carrying out a local survey of exercise participation leading to a range of other initiatives. These included group outings from one health centre for women-only swimming sessions to meet the cultural needs of particular groups, rambling for inner-city children in the Welsh mountains, and support for collaborative fun-runs with community groups to encourage community involvement and organization. From these Mersey Regional Health Authority developed a mass participation event programme in the 1980s, instigating the Liverpool Women's 10-km Run, the Liverpool–Chester–Liverpool Bike Ride and a series of North West corporate running events. All of these took place annually for over 20 years with the bike ride still an annual feature.

Other projects included the provision of occupational advice from health centres and the establishment of a Health Information Service to support the development of health promotion initiatives across the region. HART evolved over the next 30 years into an established feature of the North West public health infrastructure. 'Heart of Mersey' was established as a charity in 2005 committed to following the 'North Karelia' approach in Merseyside. This heart health charity uses local advocacy to promote national policy change in support of the health needs of its communities. As such, Heart of Mersey was part of the highly successful SmokeFree Liverpool partnership and North West collaboration which was instrumental in the successful lobbying for the Health Act in 2006, which legislated for comprehensive smoke-free enclosed public spaces.

Heart of Mersey also established the 'Healthy Stadia' initiative, working at local and international levels to promote health in partnership with sports organizations, including the European Football championships. Heart of Mersey launched 'Food Active' in 2013, a whole systems approach to addressing healthy weight in the North West, which included the first local authority declaration on healthy weight and the GULP (Give Up Loving Pop) campaign, part of the lobby for the Soft Drinks Industry Levy introduced in 2018.

Planning parenthood, learning from abroad

The discovery of the oral contraceptive pill and the rise of youth culture in the 1960s led to dramatic changes in teenage sexual behaviour. This led the poet Philip Larkin to announce in his poem 'Annus Mirabilis' that:

> Sexual intercourse began
> In nineteen sixty-three
> (which was rather late for me)—
> Between the end of the 'Chatterley' ban[1]
> And the Beatles first LP. (2)

In the United Kingdom this coincided with an era of socially liberal legislation under the government of Harold Wilson which saw the abolition of capital punishment, the loosening of laws on divorce, the legalization of homosexuality between consenting adults, and in 1967, the passing of the Abortion Act, which permitted termination of pregnancy on social grounds. One consequence of the changed environment was a shift to earlier ages of first sexual experience and an initial rise in teenage pregnancy rates in developed countries.

The rise in teenage pregnancy rates, in turn, prompted the wider availability of contraceptive services (in 1974 in England and Wales) and a falling rate of conception, which was most marked in older age groups at first, and only later among younger women. Between country comparisons of the rate of decline in teenage conception gives a good indication of the extent to which policy changes in the form of relationships education and birth control, together with youth counselling services, have been responsive to the needs of young people

---

[1] Referring to the celebrated court case over D. H. Lawrence's novel *Lady Chatterley's Lover*, which had been banned for obscenity.

and their desire to behave in a responsible way. Whereas teenage conception rates in Sweden and Denmark fell by 40 per cent between 1970 and 1986, those in England and Wales fell by only15 per cent and those in the United States actually increased.

The Wessex Abortion Studies, Gotland, and the Liverpool Project

My own involvement in this important area of public health predates the move back to Liverpool. As a young psychiatrist moving into public health I had struggled to find a topic for my Masters dissertation that would combine my clinical background with my new public health career and which combined prevention and mental health. I took advice from many senior people in psychiatry but I drew a blank. The nearest anybody could get was early diagnosis and treatment in the community, secondary, not primary prevention, in public health terms. In the end I hit on planned parenthood as something at the very foundations of good mental health and I carried out a series of studies into family planning and abortion provision in the Wessex region of the south of England, beginning in 1975. At that time the moral panic over teenage sexual behaviour, and the pregnancy rates and abortions that accompanied it, was reaching a crescendo with polarization between those who sought to understand the major societal changes that were underway and respond to them, and those who, King Canute-like, wished to push the waves back. I was greatly helped in this work by the chairman of the Wessex Regional Health Authority, Mr Kingsley Williams, and by the professor of Human Reproduction at Southampton, John Dennis, who was one of a stable of socially orientated obstetricians who had been trained in Aberdeen by the father of social obstetrics, Sir Dugald Baird.

On the face of it the issue was a straightforward one, that a large proportion of pregnant women from the Wessex Region were seeking terminations of pregnancy by travelling up to 100 difficult miles along the south coast to Brighton where they had to pay for their operations. This was in contrast to the service provided by John Dennis and his colleagues in Southampton which was readily accessible free of charge on the National Health Service. The problem was especially acute in the west of the region, in Dorset, where young women were having to sell personal possessions to pay for their treatment.

The outcome was a comprehensive set of studies which addressed the issues of patient choice, decision making and delay, the institutional and clinical factors which were preventing an equitable service, and the resultant clinical outcomes for the women involved. It transpired that the women would have overwhelmingly chosen to have had an early operation near to their homes and that young women were especially disadvantaged with both access to contraception in the first place and access to early abortion, with implications for their later health and wellbeing. The attitudes of consultant gynaecologists towards the provision of a service were critical. In a remarkable meeting of all the regions' consultant gynaecologists a set of options was proposed:

1. To put additional resources into the problem districts with the hope that this would improve the availability of operations;

2. To provide a regional day care abortion service caring for all the women in the region;

3. For the regional health authority to pay the charitable clinic to carry out the operations on the women from the region who needed to travel to Brighton; and

4. To do none of these things.

The meeting voted against all the options including doing nothing but did not propose anything else. The outcome was that the regional health authority agreed to pay the women's bills.

Lessons from Sweden—A vertical problem struggling to go horizontal

This experience galvanized my thoughts on the whole issue of teenage sexuality and relationships, and was helped along by support from the then Chief Executive of the Health Education Council in London, Dr David Player. It led to my developing a collaboration between Sweden and Liverpool with a focus on young people, their relationships, and sexuality.

Over the past 150 years and more there have been profound changes in the physical and social aspects of adolescence, the age of onset of sexual maturation has been steadily decreasing, growth and physical development have proceeded at an accelerated pace together with a trend towards greater adult size, albeit with marked social class variations in the height and weight of school leavers; the age of menarche has become much earlier against a background of better nutrition and changed economic circumstances.

In parallel with these changes the 1960s and 1970s saw massive changes in the social culture and lifestyles of teenagers, accompanied by a longer period of dependency through the extension of further and higher education with later marriage. More recently economic conditions have impacted on the millennial cohorts reaching majority after the year 2000 with implications that are only just becoming apparent. At the time that these changes were gathering momentum a number of reasons were identified as underpinning the changes in teenage sexual behaviour:

1. Changes in attitudes
2. Changes in parental behaviour
3. Rising levels of divorce
4. Lessening influence of religion
5. Influence of the media and of advertising
6. Peer group pressure.

It has also seemed that the source of young people's information about sex is important and that the more open and informative parents are about sex, the less likely teenagers are to experience early intercourse. Most people now accept that planned parenthood is an important and attainable goal. There is a considerable body of evidence to show that the birth of unplanned and unintended children is associated with major disadvantages for these children which have social, psychological, and physical dimensions. Early teenage pregnancy is associated with a variety of physical problems for the mother and with increased perinatal and maternal mortality. From the economic point of view, as measured by the costs to society of unplanned pregnancy, birth control has been shown to be extremely cost effective.

Until recently the birth of an unintended child was much more common among teenagers than among older women; some of the underlying reasons for this have involved the constellation of moral, psychological, educational, organizational, and political factors surrounding community attitudes towards sexuality, health education, and youth counselling services. In the United Kingdom we have come a long way since the 1970s but we still lag behind some other countries, in particular those in Scandinavia and the Netherlands. When a teenager marries, often as a result of pregnancy it is much less likely to endure than the marriage of an older woman.

Looking back now, what is remarkable is how significant decreases in teenage pregnancy rates have nevertheless occurred over a period when teenagers have in general become sexually active at younger ages. In the mid-1970s between a half and two-thirds of young people had had intercourse by the age of 19; today, a significant proportion have had sex by the age of 16 although there are recent suggestions that the younger generation is becoming less sexually active.

A community approach

By the 1960s Sweden was attracting attention as a liberated and socially permissive country. As a teenager hitchhiking around Europe at the age of 17, I was surprised to find condom machines prominently displayed in public places. For whatever reasons, a combination of secular and Lutheran values was in the process of trailblazing for other countries in its approach to teenage sexuality. By the early 1970s systematic approaches were being developed in more than half the Swedish counties which addressed the prevailing spiritual, public, parental, and professional dimensions of the new challenge. In this they were undoubtedly influenced by the emerging lessons from North Karelia about public engagement and the reorientation of health, social, and educational services towards public health and prevention. The focus was not only on sex education but also caring support and positive acceptance during young people's first adult relationship. As expressed by one Swede, Carl Gustav Boethius:

> when young people are blamed for going steady, they become desperate. When they have the experience of being accepted—when they feel that parents and teachers look with sympathy and joy at them and their boyfriend and girlfriend then they have the feeling 'we must take care of this, we must live up to the confidence they have in us. We would even like to discuss the situation with them and maybe even take advice from them.' (3)

This seems to be a very moral position in which adults accept their duty of care towards adolescents. Underlying such a view is an acceptance both of sexuality as a positive force in relationships and of the fact that our children are indeed 'only lent to us for a short time'.

The model which was developed in Sweden was based on the necessity of 'breaking down the conspiracy of silence between the generations' and was aimed at creating community-wide initiatives which moved and spread 'like rings on the water'. The general approach was through intensive residential workshops for key opinion formers, decision makers, role models, teachers, other professionals, and counsellors of young people. The agenda for these workshops included factual information about human biology, personal relationships and the family, pornography, prostitution, and venereal disease (this was in the pre-AIDS years). The methods used included lectures, role play, discussions, group work, theatre, and film. The intention was to provide a non-threatening learning and working environment where attitudes and values could be explored, ignorance remedied, and common ground sought.

Of particular value was found to be a short history of four generations in a farming community on the Baltic island of Gotland written by the district nurse and midwife from her own experience. This simple account of how family life had changed within living memory struck a chord with workshop participants who could set aside simple myths about the 'good old days' compared with the horrors of modern times when confronted with the realities of women having annual pregnancies in pre-contraceptive times, and where marital rape was common. This practical ethnographic narrative seemed to facilitate the creative process of finding practical solutions in a remarkable way.

Workshops like these were held around the Swedish counties, involving people at town, village, and school levels. As a result several hundred key people would, in effect become resources for programme initiatives, such as group discussions in school or the visits of teenagers to community clinics to familiarize themselves with the services which were available, and provide opportunities for seminars aimed at raising sensitivity to the need for contraception as a joint responsibility within a relationship. The mainstream work was reinforced by events such as festivals and mobile services and was carried out with the collaboration of the media from the outset. In the Gothenburg programme after two years of work, a one-week film festival was held, involving all the schools, in which the cinemas put on a constantly changing programme of films about love and sex, romance and pornography, for viewing and subsequent debate and discussion across the city and its communities and in school classrooms.

With the focus on relationships and 'living together' rather than on the mechanics of sex and contraception, the Swedish initiatives met with considerable success. Not only was there a subsequent 40 per cent reduction in teenage conception rates, but this was also accompanied by falls in sexually transmitted disease, and claims that drug abuse and delinquency were also in decline.

The Liverpool Project

Back in Liverpool, at the request of the Health Education Council, I set about trying to replicate the Swedish experience. Visits to Finland and Sweden had given me first-hand insights into the exciting new ways of approaching public health with an eclectic menu of methods that included the arts, cinema, theatre, mass media, and community development, acting on both qualitative and quantitative evidence. Initial attempts to replicate the Scandinavian experience met a mixed reception.

The population of the Liverpool health district in the early 1980s was around 500,000 with a heterogeneous demography. Strong historic links to the Republic of Ireland meant that the Roman Catholic Church was still influential with its strict views on sex outside of marriage. Nevertheless, the city had one of the highest teenage pregnancy, illegitimacy, and abortion rates in the country. Despite an extensive network of health authority family planning clinics there was no special provision of birth control and youth advisory services for young people other than a limited service provided by the Brook Advisory Centre, a charity. Provision of specialist clinics for young people had been recommended in a Department of Health memorandum which proposed 'separate, less formal arrangements for young people. The staff should be experienced in dealing with young people and their problems' (4). This was something which the Dutch had pursued vigorously since the early 1970s with dramatic impact.

The proposal for a community-based intervention to address the problem in Liverpool was commissioned by the Health Education Council in London in 1983. During the next three years a process which took account of the Swedish experience was followed. These attempts to develop a demonstration project which would be acceptable to both the Health Education Council and its paymaster, a socially conservative government, has also to be seen against a continuing controversy over the liberalization of abortion access and a focus on the prescribing of oral contraceptives to girls under the age of 16 years. This focus had led to a test case brought by Mrs Victoria Gillick to the House of Lords in 1984 in which Mrs Gillick had sought to establish that under no circumstances would any of her daughters (Beatrice, Hannah, Jessie, or Sarah) be given contraceptive or abortion treatment while they were under 16 in any local health authority family planning clinic, without her prior knowledge and irrefutable evidence of her consent.

Having failed to obtain the assurances which she required, Mrs Gillick began legal proceedings against her local health authority. In July 1983 she lost her case in the High Court and began to contest the ruling in the Court of Appeal. In December 1984 her appeal was upheld in the following terms:

> That the notice (of guidance) issued by the department (of Health) . . . is contrary to Law. That no Doctor or other professional person employed by the first defendants . . . may give contraceptive and/or abortion advice to any child of the plaintiff below the age of 16 without the prior knowledge and/or consent of the said child's parent or guardian save in cases of emergency, or with the leave of the court. (5)

There followed a period of almost 12 months of extreme uncertainty. Youth advisory clinics reported a dramatic reduction in the numbers of younger teenagers seeking contraceptive advice, and family planning nurses reported that they had been prohibited from teaching in schools. An acrimonious debate was waged through the media with the political right proclaiming the death of the permissive society and sexual health workers and health educators struggling to mobilize middle-of-the-road opinion to defend long fought-for freedoms. This fight took place over the heads of the teenagers affected: the moralists against the professionals and the politically committed. The real losers in this were those teenagers who were becoming newly sexually active and who, temporarily at least, had lost access to those services which were controlled by adults. Finally, the Law Lords ruled by two to one against Mrs Gillick, supporting the Department of Health appeal against the Appeal Court ruling of December 1984.

In initiating a process of consultation in Liverpool, prior to a project, an understanding of the potential pitfalls was central to the consultation strategy adopted. It was essential to establish a relationship based on trust between key community representatives, decision makers, and professionals, to secure the cooperation of people with different belief systems for the common good. After taking advice from local senior public health officials and being told it was a waste of time trying to engage with the Catholic schools, I found the opposite to be the case and that the late Bishop Worlock and his head of school pastoral affairs, Father Vincent Nichols, could not have been more helpful. In taking the line that all Catholic schools should have sex education, the explanation that 'of course they should have it, because if they don't, how will they know it's wrong when we tell them?' (6), was more than enough to work with. The helpful and enlightened Vincent Nichols went on to become a Roman Catholic Cardinal.

The most important initial work included the development of a structured consultation to establish prevailing attitudes among community representatives, decision makers, and professionals towards teenage pregnancy and sexually transmitted disease, to establish whether there was support for a project and, if so, what the constraints and facilitating factors would be. A wide network of contacts and people committed to some sort of intervention was identified, including:

1. Young people, self-help, and women's groups, and groups with special needs such as homosexuals;

2. Representatives of ethnic minorities;

3. Religious bodies (the Church of England, the Roman Catholic Church, and the Jewish Synagogue);

4. Specific service providers for young people (counselling and guidance clinics both statutory and voluntary);

5. Youth and community workers;

6. Social services for young people including specialist services, child care, fostering, and intermediate treatment;

7. Education workers (teachers, advisers, school inspectors, parent support, and teacher trainers); and

8. Medical and nursing personnel, including those from obstetrics, genitourinary medicine, paediatrics, public health, general practice, and family planning.

In all about 50 people became involved and provided the basis for a three-day residential workshop conducted along lines developed by the Swedish Board of Health, with the assistance of the British Family Planning Association

Education Unit and resource people from China and Sweden. The workshop consisted of small and large group sessions with the following objectives:

1. To make explicit the values of the participants;
2. To match these values against participants' perceptions of the needs of young people;
3. To identify whether there would be general support for a demonstration project and to clarify the nature of such a project; and
4. To identify those factors which might facilitate or hinder the success of such a project.

Analysis of the feedback from the workshop participants identified three essential sub-programmes of a demonstration project:

1. Education and training for interpersonal relationships, probably based on the Swedish model;
2. Socio-health services for young people; and
3. Information and media resources.

In addition a research agenda was identified to support action, and specific recommendations which took account of the special position taken by the Roman Catholic Archdiocese in identifying areas of common concern and agreement were made. This included, in particular, the willingness of the archdiocese to cooperate in working to enhance and deepen personal relationships among teenagers and a statement supporting a programme of sex education in Liverpool schools. There was agreement about the desire to work against the exploitation of sexuality in the media and in advertising, to reduce the number of induced abortions among teenagers, and to eradicate sexually transmitted disease. Differences between people on these issues concerned means rather than ends. One outcome of the collaboration with the faith communities was the invitation to participate in a series of regular seminars held with active lay members of the Roman Catholic Church. The highlight of one of these sessions, attended by over 200 people in a cordial spirit, was when the father of teenage girls proclaimed that 'we have to tell young people the good news about sex'.

The importance of not seeing teenage sexuality in isolation from the overall condition of young people, or of viewing young people as a problem was implicit in many of the discussions at this time. When it comes to teenage sex we have often been caught in a web of our own making. Family planning professionals can sometimes appear to be motivated primarily by paternalistic and hygienist considerations rather than by the quest for autonomy and authenticity, with its implication that people are trusted to make informed choices for themselves. The dilemma of health is well put by the savage in his conversation with Mustapha Mond in Huxley's *Brave New World*:

'I want poetry, I want freedom, I want goodness, I want sin.

'In fact', said Mustapha Mond (from the new world), 'you're claiming the right to be unhappy'.

'Not to mention the right to grow old and ugly and impotent; the right to have syphilis and cancer; the right to have little to eat; the right to be lousy; the right to live in constant apprehension of what may happen tomorrow; the right to catch typhoid; the right to be tortured by unspeakable pains of every kind!'

There was a long silence.

'I claim them all', said the savage at last.

Mustapha Mond shrugged his shoulders. 'You're welcome to them', he said. (7)

In January 1986 the proposal for a demonstration project in Liverpool was rejected by the Health Education Council despite three years' work, the expenditure of time, money, and the goodwill of a community of half a million people. The position still being taken, with the threat of HIV/AIDS beginning to become significant, was still very much as 'the ostrich position', with heads buried in the sand. Within months that was all about to change as the new epidemic began to unfold. Meanwhile the groundwork that we had done for the Liverpool Project would pay off in less direct ways; the community of Liverpool had begun to talk about sex, and the statistics would reflect the benefit of this over the coming years. Of immediate importance would be the interagency collaboration in the face of the combined threat of injecting drug use and the spread of the AIDS virus.

The Guttmacher report on teenage pregnancy in developed countries

As the 1980s progressed and as the baby boomers came of age and began to give voice to more liberal attitudes together with the changed imperatives brought on by the AIDS epidemic, the climate of public opinion began to change. One of the turning points was the publication in 1986 of a major international study of teenage pregnancy in 37 developed countries by the independent Alan Guttmacher Institute in New York, with which I was privileged to be a collaborator. The study was carried out in two stages: the first was a statistical comparison of teenage sexual behaviour and pregnancy in 37 countries, the second an in-depth, qualitative examination of the situation in the United States, and five approximately comparable countries illustrative of the range of teenage pregnancy rates. An enormous range in these annual rates was identified from 14 per thousand 15–19 year olds in the Netherlands to 96 per thousand in the

United States with Sweden (35), France (43), Canada (44), and England and Wales (45), being somewhere in the middle. The differences could not be explained by variations in sexual activity among the teenagers of the different countries or by greater recourse to abortion. Rather it seemed that all other things being equal the teenagers in the different countries varied in the effectiveness with which they used contraception.

The Guttmacher researchers concluded that there seemed to be three major determinants of this effectiveness:

1. The degree of openness about sexuality and the extent of acceptance of teenage sexuality by the adult community;

2. The availability of good quality information and education about sexual matters; and

3. The provision of high-quality, user-friendly clinical services for young people.

The Guttmacher report appeared at the same time that the AIDS epidemic was galvanizing the world to focus on sexual health, and it received massive publicity internationally. One reporter, Irene Sege of the *Boston Globe*, focused in on the issue of openness and acceptance of teenage sexuality and visited Europe to explore for herself the differences from the United States. In Amsterdam she spent two weeks in many small group discussions with teenagers, their parents, and teachers before travelling to Liverpool where I arranged for her to repeat the exercise. At the end of her research Irene reported to me in a personal communication that 'the difference between Amsterdam and Liverpool is quite clear, in Amsterdam parents talk with their children about sex'.

All change, all systems go

In the early 1980s when the Liverpool project was being mooted, it was common to find managers who were unsympathetic to teenage sexuality and who often censored the list of possible solutions on the basis that parents or perhaps the church might object and cause them difficulties. In fact the overwhelming majority of parents in the UK expected their children to receive sex and relationships education at school, and were sympathetic to the provision of youth advisory services which included contraception. Furthermore the climate of opinion was steadily strengthening as the 1960s generation became adults and parents, and the practicalities of responding to the threat of HIV/AIDS and the need to talk about safe sex became apparent. Nevertheless it would take another 30 years before the British government took the decision to make sex and relationships education compulsory in all schools including faith-based and private institutions.

In Liverpool and the North West, however, we had the benefit of strong and progressive leadership in the form of chairman of the regional health authority, Sir Donald Wilson, who had already demonstrated his metal by supporting the provision of the first large-scale syringe exchange programme despite government reluctance in 1986. The opportunity to take strategic action finally dawned in 1991 with the publication of a public health Green Paper by the Thatcher Government when it fell to me to present the proposals to each of the district health authorities and finally to the regional health authority itself.

It was at this point that my longstanding interest in planned parenthood and abortion, which had begun in Wessex 14 years previously, finally began to pay off.

The Green Paper, as the basis for legislation, had no mention of the topic which was so close to my heart so I took the opportunity of introducing it in the discussion with the health authorities. Years of work, of monitoring the statistics, and of seeing the power of the Karelia and the Guttmacher summary data led me to a succinct summary of the local position at that time which I was able to share:

♦ Every year out of every 1000 16- to 19-year-old Liverpool women, 81 became pregnant, of whom 24 would have an abortion, 50 would have a child without being married, and 7 would become married with poor prospects for the union enduring.

I presented this data to the regional health authority on the Tuesday; on the Thursday I ran into the Authority Chief Executive who told me of the disturbing effect it had had on the Chairman: 'He couldn't sleep that night, he phoned me up but we couldn't find your phone number , you had better phone him up on the farm'. Eventually I got through to Sir Donald on the farm and his response was short and to the point, if not politically correct; 'Isn't there something we can do like we did with the junkies?' The outcome was a meeting the following week which lasted for one hour and produced a ten-point action plan with allocated responsibilities.

The implementation of this plan began immediately, anticipating the government's inclusion of sexual health in the 'Health of the Nation', and the much more systematic approach adopted by the Blair government after 1997. Guidelines were drawn up for discussion with schools and education authorities as to what should be happening, and an agenda-setting conference of all head teachers was held at Everton Football Club. Systematic refocusing of clinical services was undertaken which shifted resources away from clinics for older and married women who were now able to access birth control from family doctors and nurses, reinvesting it in youth provision. A specialist family planning clinic was established for older women with special contraceptive needs which became a centre of excellence for research and training. Six specially chosen family doctor practices were identified on a geographic basis where the physicians had a special interest in sexual health and they were each allocated a family planning nurse made possible by the reconfiguration of clinics.

Until this point the charitable Brook Advisory Clinic, providing contraceptive advice to young people, had been struggling along from hand to mouth in unsatisfactory first floor premises above a city centre shop. One morning the regional health authority chairman appeared in the office having made an unsolicited field visit to Brook the previous evening. With queues of young people extending down the stairs and out on to the pavement, boyfriends as well as girlfriends, Sir Donald was more than satisfied that this was what young people wanted and what we should support. A significant increase in funding followed and during the next few years the client base grew rapidly from 1000 patients each year to over 30,000 with a concomitant impact on unplanned teen pregnancy rates.

Following the change of national government in 1997, I was fortunate in working closely with the new Minister of Public Health, Dame Tessa Jowell, and Chief Medical Officer Sir Liam Donaldson in drafting a New Public Health strategy for England. Embedded within this was a major initiative on teenage pregnancy which was in no small measure influenced by our work in Liverpool and the North West. As Winston Churchill was reputed to have said of the Americans 'The Americans always do the right thing, having tried everything else first'. Finally Parliament, the dispensary of public health had spoken. Today, over 30 years since the Guttmacher report, teenage pregnancy rates in England and Wales are half what they were in 1986; however, they are still more than twice the rates of those in Scandinavia and the Netherlands.

Asset-based community development— the example of the Eldon Street Community Association

When John McKnight assumed the mantle of the legendary Chicago community organizer Saul Alinsky at the Center for Urban Affairs at Northwestern University, he and his colleagues focused their research on urban neighbourhoods. The outcome of this work and of 4000 doorstep interviews which asked the question 'What has happened around here recently to make a difference?' was the formulation of an understanding of neighbourhoods focused on the usefulness of local resources, capacities, and relationships. This work was documented in a guide entitled 'Building Communities from the Inside Out', which described an approach to community building based on mapping the assets, human, environmental, and social that can be identified in any community however disadvantaged. This book became a major influence internationally in the subsequent years.

The five components of a map of community assets as identified by McKnight and his colleagues can be represented visually (Box 4.1).

Key ideas at the heart of asset-based community development include the notions that 'individuals and communities are half full rather than half empty', that 'it takes a village to raise a child', and that 'you don't go to the store until you have seen what you have in your back yard'. Early in his career McKnight had worked with Ivan Illich, the author of *Medical Nemesis* and *Deschooling Society*, in South America and carried with him the conviction that professionals must learn to operate in different ways if they were to be part of the solution rather than part of the problem. Although I was aware of John McKnight's work on my return to Liverpool in 1982, I did not have the privilege of meeting and working with him until much later when I was working in Cumbria. Nevertheless his ideas fell on fertile soil when I came into contact with the Eldon Street Community Association in the old Irish district of north Liverpool.

Eldon Street is situated in the Liverpool local government ward of Vauxhall, half a mile north of the city centre in the heart of the city's dockland and until after the Second World War it had been an area of remarkably high-density slum housing. During the early years of the twentieth century many of the slum courts, familiar to Dr Duncan, had been demolished and replaced with the first social or council housing in England. The German Luftwaffe with its blitzkrieg of the Liverpool docks in 1941 and the wholesale slum clearance of the 1960s led to further remodelling and thinning out, with thousands of families being compulsorily rehoused to new estates on the edge of the city. Friends and neighbours were split up and social networks destroyed. The disruption was widely held by local people to have led to the premature death of many elderly people.

Box 4.1 The components of a community asset map

An instigator
Associations
Institutions
Environments
Gappers or Connectors who facilitate the relationships of the other
  components.

In 1978, the first the community knew about a further round of demolition was when letters dropped through the letterboxes one morning producing a general sense of shock and trepidation. What followed was remarkable. Local parish priest Father Dunn convened a community meeting, introduced it, and stood back; the anger of the local people was channelled into a fight against what seemed destined to befall them. 'Yes' they wanted new houses, but they had no intention of allowing further traumas to afflict their neighbourhoods. They wanted new houses to replace the old and in the same area. The Eldon Street Community Association (motto 'We do it better ourselves') was formed with a street-based committee structure and the local people set about fighting for the right to be rehoused locally. They conducted their own surveys of people's housing wishes and began to develop their own plans in collaboration with local housing associations, socially orientated architects, and, once I had become involved, with the local universities and regional health authority.

In 1982 this community, which was already greatly stressed, received a body blow when the Tate and Lyle sugar refinery, the major local employer, closed with the loss of 2000 jobs. This was part of a more general disaster for Merseyside as companies abandoned their historic northern roots and headed for London and the south east to be closer to the new markets offered by Europe. Thousands of other jobs in port-related work were lost in the space of several years and the adult male unemployment rate rose above 50 per cent.

We know that unsatisfactory housing can affect health in a variety of ways. We are also now aware of the strong and significant associations between unemployment and both mental and physical ill-health. In the case of mental illness the causal nature of these associations has been established beyond doubt. The range of mental health problems identified includes depression, para-suicide, and suicide itself. As with physical health, the incidence of problems increases with the duration of unemployment. The range of physical disorders includes heart disease, chronic bronchitis, lung cancer, and infant growth retardation. In 1980s Merseyside an epidemic of heroin abuse was waiting in the wings for alienated and disaffected youth; a veritable modern cholera equivalent.

In Vauxhall, housing, environmental, economic, and social stress converged to produce the worst health in the city at the time; standardized mortality ratios were 50 per cent higher than those for England and Wales; more than two-thirds of children were in receipt of free school meals; a ratio of 1 in 200 school leavers went to further education compared with 1 in 5 in the affluent areas—all these give an indication of the enormity of the challenge. For the community itself its priority was housing and then jobs. Although health was of concern and our collaboration was beginning to reveal the extent of the health divide with others in the city, action on health would have to wait until more fundamental issues were addressed. (See Box 4.2.)

The Vauxhall community based on Eldon Street had a strong belief in the importance of a sense of place in their own wellbeing, an understanding which is too often overlooked by bureaucracies in planning services. Drawing on the strength of its geographical roots and the traditional cultural cohesion of its church links, this community was on a journey of taking control over its own destiny. Over 30 years later it can point to a long string of community initiatives for which it has been responsible: from extensive housing cooperatives, community-owned businesses, and services for its elderly residents to the regeneration of tracts of derelict land into green space and sports and community facilities. Such was the success at transforming the image and reputation of the area that in time it became a safe bet for private house builders to appear and build houses for sale, not uncommonly being bought by those who had been compulsorily rehoused far away many years before.

And in due course we began to address the health issues. During the worst of the drug epidemic years of the 1980s and 1990s the community cohesion meant that drug dealers knew that they were unwelcome locally and Vauxhall avoided the worst of the blight. Questions began to be asked about the poor access to healthy food choices with a limited choice of outlets for fresh fruit and vegetables and healthy options; in time a modern supermarket was encouraged to locate in the neighbourhood; and concern about the rudimentary nature of primary health care resulted in capital being found to rebuild a run-down health centre. Not only did the community association have equal time with the professionals in working with the architects but they also appointed their own family doctors, living evidence of their philosophy that professionals should be

Box 4.2 Dealing with the elephants

There is a story about an agency in Asia going into a village with very high infant mortality from gastroenteritis and diarrhoeal disease, and constructing latrines without consulting the village elders as to their own priorities. On returning 2 years later, they found the latrines unused. At this point the community was consulted and it was found that their priority was the elephants. Every year the elephants would trample down the sugar just when it was nearly ripe and the village lost a major part of its potential income. The agency now cooperated with the villagers in finding ways to keep the elephants out. Later they began to discuss sanitation.

'on tap not on top'. This was very much a two-way learning process which recognized McKnight's criticism of welfare programmes in which the majority of budgets benefit professionals rather than the poor, with money passing through communities without touching the sides.

The asset-based approach found its form in the way in which professionals who became involved with the Eldonians began to work as coaches, facilitators, and connectors. Mapping of the cash flows through the ward was undertaken to better understand how it might be put to the use of the local people; the treasurers department of the regional health authority was put to use as a banker for large sums of social investment moneys until the community had the confidence and skills to assume its own financial control, and assistance was given by various agencies in the arcane business of writing funding proposals.

Years later people who had no formal education after they left school can look back with satisfaction on the way they took back control of their own community and created a brighter future, and better health and wellbeing for their children and grandchildren.

Evaluation

The evaluation of whole system interventions as comprehensive as that in Vauxhall is not easy. On one level the major questions are about reducing the inequalities in mortality and ill-health compared with other parts of the city, but even this is not straightforward. With increased wellbeing and better life chances comes increased social mobility, and difficulties in comparing like with like, with outcomes that may only take place over two or three generations. Yet most academic approaches to evaluation are limited to a time scale of several years and a reductionist focus on specific single-factor cause-and-effect relationships. Within health service systems there is a strong emphasis on value for money and on measures of efficiency; effectiveness and health outcomes are rarely addressed.

Even in celebrated large-scale public health interventions such as the Karelia Project or the Swedish teenage pregnancy work it is difficult to claim credit for an intervention in achieving an effect, against a backcloth of massive trends in behaviour change. Five strands appear to be necessary for evaluation research in modern public health:

1. The need for positive indicators in place of negative ones and for qualitative and small area data;
2. The need to focus on contexts as well as people;
3. Doing things from where people are: people- and community-centred perspectives;

4. The need for true stories; and

5. Assessment of the health promoting assets of communities.

References

1. **Chave, S. P. W.**, *Recalling the Medical Officer of Health: writings*, ed. **Michael Warren** and **Huw Francis**. London: King Edwards Hospital Fund for London, 1987.

2. **Larkin, Philip**, 'Annus Mirabilis', in *High Windows*. London: Faber, 1974.

3. **National Board of Health and Welfare**, *Committee on Health Education Living Together—A Family Planning Project on Gotland Sweden 1973-76*. Sweden: National Board of Health and Welfare, 1978.

4. **Laing, W. A.**, *Family Planning: the Benefits and Costs*. London: Policy Studies Institute, 1982.

5. **Stocking, B.**, *Initiative and Inertia: Case Studies in the N.H.S.* London : Nuffield Provincial Hospitals Trust, 1985.

6. **Ashton, John**, and **Howard Seymour**, *The New Public Health*. Oxford: Oxford University Press, 1988.

7. **Huxley, Aldous**. *Brave New World*, pp. 211–12. London: Penguin Random House, 2007.

Further Reading

Ashton. J. R., The experiences of women refused N.H.S. abortion. *J. Bio-social Science* (1980), **12**: 201–10.

Community Control of Cardiovascular Diseases: North Karelia Project. Copenhagen: National Public Health Laboratory Finland, Regional Office of World Health Organization.

Dennis, J., Draper, P., Griffiths, J., Partridge, J., Popay, J., and **others**, *Rethinking Community Medicine: Unit for the Study of Health Policy*. London: Guys Hospital, 1979.

Hussey, R. M., M. B. Edwards, J. A. Reid, K. Sykes, H. Seymour, E. Hopley, J. R. Ashton, Evaluation of the International Garden Festival Health Fair. *Public Health* (1987), 111–17.

Jones, Elise F., Jacqueline Darroch Forrest, Noreen Goldman, Stanley K. Henshaw, Richard Lincoln, Jennie I. Rosoff, Charles Westoff, and **Deidre Wulf**, Teenage pregnancy in developed countries: determinants and policy implications. *Family Planning Perspectives* (1985), **17**: 53–63.

Kretzmann, John P., and **John L. McKnight**, *Building Communities from the Inside Out: A Path toward Finding and Mobilizing a Community's Assets*. Evanston, IL: Asset-Based Community Development Institute, 1993.

Lalonde, M., *A New Perspective on the Health of Canadians*. Minister of Supply and Services Canada, 1974.

Larson, B., *A Gotland Family*, ed. Hanna Olsson. Stockholm: National Swedish Board of Health and Welfare, 1975.

McBane, Jack, *The Rebirth of Liverpool: The Eldonian Way*. Liverpool: Liverpool University Press, 2008.

McKnight, John, *The Careless Society: Community and its Counterfeits*. New York: Basic Books, 1995.

McKnight, John, and Peter Block. *The Abundant Community, Awakening the Power of Families and Neighbourhoods*. San Francisco: American Planning Association, Barrett-Koehler Publishers, 2010.

Titmuss, R. M., *Social Policy—An Introduction*. London: George Allen and Unwin, 1974.

World Health Organization, Health and Welfare Canada, and Canadian Public Health Association, *The Ottawa Charter for Health Promotion*. Copenhagen: WHO, 1986.

Chapter 5

Protecting health

Protecting the health of the population against external threats lies at the heart of public health and is a fundamental function of government. In Germany, Neumann had put it succinctly in 1847, when arguments were raging between free marketeers who believed in a minimalist State, and those who wanted intervention on behalf of the poor and vulnerable:

> The State argues that its responsibility is to protect people's property rights. For most people the only property which they possess is their health; therefore the State has a responsibility to protect people's health. (1)

This may seem obvious when it comes to the threat of inter-country war and violence, but the responsibility for prevention for the wide range of other external threats may be contested until being brought into focus at times of acute incident or emergency. However, governments that are unsighted on issues that might jump up and bite them do so at their peril. What might start as an episode or incident has a habit of turning without warning into an emergency or a disaster. It is at this point that the public begins to ask questions and point fingers.

Health protection and the determinants of health

The classic triad of disease was long defined as the interaction between agent, host, and environment in which microbes were the dominant agent mediating between biology and the outside world. Today we are more likely to identify genetic/biological, environmental, lifestyle/behavioural, and technical interventions as the major influences on health and wellbeing, and include economic/social and psychological factors. We now understand that it is artificial to compartmentalize these dimensions because they interact, and in searching for unity we find that policies for health and health care have the potential to be cross cutting.

In 1979, the United States Surgeon General, in his ground-breaking report 'Healthy People', drew the distinction between preventive health care, health protection, and health promotion based on a set of health goals for healthy infants and children, healthy adults, and healthy older people. This had the advantage of combining a lifecycle approach with one which categorized the scope of public health work by the determinants of health and disease (see Box 5.1).

One of the World Health Organization's most significant contributions to health development has been the Healthy Cities project and the focus on settings and place which it has generated. Settings such as schools, workplaces, prisons, sports stadia, hospitals, and neighbourhoods have been identified as tangible environments in which the determinants of health can be considered, and where policies, programmes, and projects for health protection and improvement can be made meaningful and grounded.

Box 5.1 US Surgeon General's Healthy People Framework

Preventive health services

- Family planning
- Pregnancy and infant care
- Immunization
- Sexually transmitted disease
- High blood pressure control

Health promotion

- Smoking cessation
- Reducing misuse of alcohol and drugs
- Improved nutrition
- Exercise and fitness
- Stress control

Health protection

- Toxic agent control
- Occupational health and safety
- Accidental injury control
- Fluoridation of community water supplies
- Infectious disease control

Making health protection real

The value of health protection as a concept is in its focus on the more external threats to public health. It has become important to distinguish this from traditional environmental health which had become identified with a narrow range of technical tasks undertaken by a specific cadre of workers acting within a particular legal framework. In contrast, today's external and environmental threats to health are more complex, more global and diffuse and frequently require whole system responses. They go beyond the specifics of infectious disease, important as these remain, require an ecological rather than a sanitary orientation, and are not within the gift of one group or agency. They demand dynamic partnerships including those with the public and responses that are integrated both horizontally and vertically. So where do we start? How about Chapter 20 of the *International Classification of Diseases*? (see Box 5.2)

If we include in this list communicable diseases together with a wider range of food, water, and air issues we have a frame of reference with which to organize ourselves and our work in public health and an extensive agenda to address. To be effective we must have a strategic approach and a road map with a set of arrangements that are fit for purpose. This requires technical expertise in a range of disciplines going well beyond the traditional biological laboratories to include environmental epidemiology, the social sciences, risk assessment, risk management, and risk communication. Full public engagement is essential.

My suggestion for a definition of health protection might therefore be:

> [T]he organised efforts of citizens, their representatives and experts to protect human health from external threats in ways which do not threaten the habitat of future generations and which take special measures to protect those most at risk.

In the late 1990s we moved towards this concept in the North West of England by bringing together the component disciplines of health protection

Box 5.2 Chapter 20 of the *International Statistical Classification of Diseases and Related Health Problems* (WHO)

'[G]uns, drowning, cars, machines, electricity, radiation, chemicals, smoke, fire, flames, heat, venom, earthquakes, volcanoes, war, poison, dehydration, starvation, self-harm, drugs, alcohol, assault (including sexual), riots, sharp objects, blunt objects, falls and the unintended consequences of medical care'. (2)

as one function. In doing this, we had anticipated the cataclysmic events of 11 September 2001, in New York, when the twin towers of the World Trade Centre were destroyed by terrorists and the spotlight fell on the arrangements for health protection around the world. In the United Kingdom the reboot of functions under the Health Protection Agency failed to make the transition from the biological and chemical laboratory to the whole system. Its successor, Public Health England, has struggled to escape the constraints of government, to become the truly independent voice of public health and health protection that the public needs and deserves if we are to be prepared for the unthinkable.

On the spectrum of challenges from incident to disaster it is customary to distinguish between the 'slow burn' (e.g. bovine spongiform encephalopathy); the 'rising tide' (e.g. HIV/AIDS), and the 'big bang' (e.g. a transport disaster or terrorist incident). Each of these has its own 'battle rhythm' as the incident unfolds, is recognized and responded to, perhaps by the declaration of a major incident. In this case a gold command multiagency response will be convened, usually by a chief constable (in the case of the United Kingdom). The final phase is that of recovery which may take days, weeks, and sometimes years.

Something in the water

Phenol (a big chemical bang)

On Friday 27 January 1984, 2 million people living in Merseyside, Cheshire, and North Wales awoke to find that their drinking water tasted like the antiseptic trichlorophenol (TCP). Rapidly, the rumour spread throughout the region that the supply had been sabotaged by Welsh Nationalists. Irate consumers jammed the telephone switchboards of the North West and Welsh Water authorities and the local media. Initially there was no information as to the nature of the pollution and no advice to consumers as to what they should do.

The first official explanation given was that water supplies had been affected by thawing snow with extra chlorine being added to the water at the treatment works. By the Saturday, with growing public concern, North West Water had changed its story and claimed that the water from the mountain lakes of North Wales had been polluted by phenol from an unknown source. The public was told that it was harmless but that the taste might take two days to clear from the supply. This failed to relieve the anxieties of many people and the Royal Liverpool Hospital had to call in a tanker with pure water to use for patients on renal dialysis; processed food companies suspended production and shops on Merseyside sold out of bottled water.

Throughout the weekend the picture remained unclear. Amid sporadic reports of people feeling unwell the official advice from the water authorities was that the contaminated supplies presented no threat to public health. The public response to this advice was one of growing scepticism and alarm. By the Monday, with no further information forthcoming, anxieties about the water safety were dismissed by the water authorities as 'speculation beyond your wildest dreams', whilst three local members of Parliament tabled questions in the House of Commons and called for a public inquiry. It subsequently transpired that the pollution had actually occurred at the beginning of the previous week when a tanker had discharged 200 gallons of pure phenol into the water supply and subsequently the company involved was hit with a heavy fine.

Using the University Department of Public Health as a credible platform, a public seminar was held to explore all the issues involved. When the full story emerged, it turned out that Welsh Water had known about the incident for two days before the public had been told about it but had decided that it was a historic incident and that there was no need to notify anybody else. However, a public health survey that we conducted found that almost 33 per cent of the residents of contaminated areas experienced gastrointestinal symptoms compared with 9 per cent of the residents of non-contaminated areas over the same time period. It appeared that the water authorities' definition of a threat to public health was restricted to one in which a death was likely. In fact the European Economic Community maximum permitted level for phenols in drinking water at the time was 0.0005 mg/l compared with actual levels of at least 1.5 mg/l, the long-term effects of chronic low-dose exposure to chlorophenols being unknown.

Cryptosporidium (an intermittent slow burn)

In 1989 water supplies in England and Wales were privatized under the government of Margaret Thatcher. If there was any hope that the water undertakings would become more accountable it was to be short-lived. In the early years of the new millennium, each spring several hundred people living in the area of Greater Manchester supplied with water from the Thirlmere reservoir in Cumbria became infected with cryptosporidium. 'Crypto' is present throughout the world and ranks as a leading cause of a particularly unpleasant diarrhoeal disease. It has several features that make it difficult to eliminate from water supplies being spread by oocysts that are very small and resistant to chlorine. Elimination is achieved by passing water through an adequate physical barrier such as sand filtration or a membrane less than one micron in diameter or by boiling the water.

In the case of the Thirlmere, the water is derived from feeder streams in the English Lake District which pass through fields used by grazing sheep. These pose a particular hazard during the lambing season as 'crypto' is primarily a disease of newborn lambs. The Thirlmere water is carried by a hundred mile aqueduct to Manchester, an aqueduct which was in poor condition and liable to inward leakage at various points from agricultural land along its route. A particularly bad outbreak in 1999 could be clearly tied down to the water supply from Thirlmere when comparisons were made with areas of the North West receiving water from elsewhere. United Utilities, the company providing water across the region since privatization, had a programme to renew the aqueduct but it was to take 7 years. Following public pressure from myself as Regional Director of Public Health, the timescale for remedial works was reduced to 4 years with dramatic subsequent reduction in the incidence of human infection. This example of public health advocacy illustrates the power of a trusted voice in influencing measures to protect the public even in the absence of direct control. It is salutary to reflect that in the days of the Medical Officers of Health when water was supplied by local authorities rather than private water undertakings, the Medical Officer of Health would have had a seat at the table and a responsibility to go with it.

The AIDS years—mass youth unemployment, heroin on the streets, and the HIV virus arrives—a perfect storm (rising tide)

When I had produced 'Health in Mersey' in 1984, one line was given over to the problem of narcotic abuse in the region. Within a year I was to provide evidence to the House of Commons Social Services Committee that 'very considerable concern has been expressed within this region in respect of young people and the abuse of drugs over the past 18 months'. In the meantime the local economy had tanked, generating very high levels of youth unemployment, and large quantities of heroin had begun to appear on the streets of Liverpool and the surrounding areas. HIV/AIDS was about to make its appearance. In my evidence to the committee I rehearsed a public health analysis of the situation facing us in which I argued that we needed a comprehensive approach to youth policy that would 'enable healthy teenagers to become healthy adults through enhancement of self-confidence and self-respect and an involvement with the wider community. Such a strategy must involve the commitment of the Government to youth employment, education and recreation, and involve the collaboration of central and local government and statutory and voluntary agencies in producing policies for youth' (3). In the interim we would need to provide drug treatment services to respond to the casualties produced by the failure of youth policy. Those services would evolve into the first large-scale example of a syringe exchange programme internationally and pave the way for a model of working with behavioural public health issues that would come to be known as 'Harm Reduction'.

A message from America

Liverpool was one of a number of cities to experience a heroin epidemic in the early 1980s, the situation becoming particularly acute that it became known as 'smack city'. Whereas historically narcotic abuse had been associated with access to drugs by health care professionals, increasingly an illicit trade had developed at street level. A first wave of this had occurred during the late 1960s when outbreaks of heroin abuse had been described in the south of England as conforming to an infectious disease model with describable spread from one user to another. By the 1980s so widespread was the availability of cheap heroin and increasingly other narcotics, that such a model was inadequate to explain what had become a mass threat to public health. A slow burn had become a rising tide; for the first time there were clear links between heroin use and unemployment and deprivation. The initial official response to this new situation was a hardline moral position which demanded abstinence in the face of large numbers of people in adverse social circumstances struggling with vicious addiction.

In the face of this, our response on Merseyside was to develop, with echoes of the Health of Towns Association, an alliance of key players from different sectors at the highest levels. We were in a position to do this in part because of the preparatory work we had undertaken with teenage pregnancy and the Liverpool Project. In addition to myself and the public health Team, that alliance included our chairman Sir Donald Wilson, local church leaders of different faiths together with local senior police officers, and the editor of the *Liverpool Post* and *Echo* newspapers.

With this alliance in place, the first key pieces of the jigsaw that became the Mersey Model of Harm Reduction were created. In 1985 Regional Health Promotion Officer Howard Seymour and I had met Glen Margo, the San Francisco Director of Health Education, at a public health conference in Dublin. Glen, a gay man who we later learned to be HIV+, had firsthand experience of the tsunami of AIDS that was hitting the gay community around the world. We invited Glen to Liverpool to advise us on the steps we should take to get ahead of the curve of the epidemic and he willingly obliged. Over a two-week period he ran workshops morning, afternoon, and evening with health professionals, educators, bureaucrats, personnel managers, and everybody in the city who needed to be on top of the issue. At the end of his visit we asked Glen what measures would have benefited the public health response most at the beginning of the new disease in 1979/80. Glen persuaded us that the most effective actions they had taken in San Francisco usually involved the direct engagement of the people most at risk and that near the top of that list, apart from the extensive work with gay men, would have been the provision of clean injecting equipment to drug users.

On the initiative of the church leaders, Sir Donald Wilson agreed to set up the new Mersey Drug Training and Information Centre. Numerous others were involved, including psychiatrist Dr John Marks who still followed the British approach to the treatment of drug problems recommended by the 1926 Rolleston Committee. This had endorsed the prescribing of opiate drugs in certain circumstances to those addicted to them in contrast to the dogmatic opposition to such an approach adopted by many in the psychiatric establishment. The position we took was to prove critical in the months and years ahead. With the aim of involving the people most affected, a charismatic educator and former drug addict was appointed as the Centre's Director and he went on to set up a syringe exchange programme based on some early experience in Amsterdam. Following promises from the police not to deter clients from using it, the service was set up in a low-key way in the spring of 1986, being promoted by word of mouth rather than by advertising. The editor of the *Liverpool Echo* was briefed on what was happening and agreement reached that no story would be run until we were ready when the newspaper would be able to report it exclusively. With heroin rampantly available on the streets it was not a moment too soon.

Harm reduction, heroin, and AIDS—the Mersey Model

From the outset we set three guiding principles for the Mersey Model:

1. Make contact with the whole population at risk, not just the few already in contact with health care services. We believed that this was much more likely if we provided services that were user-friendly and non-judgmental. These were provided from anonymous street-level premises in an informal setting.

2. Maintain contact. By developing therapeutic relationships with our clients over the course of time they would be more likely to make changes in their drug-taking behaviour and to stay safe from the HIV virus. In the meantime there was a good chance of avoiding other drug-related harm and keeping them in reasonable health.

3. Make changes as and when they were ready on the basis of therapeutic relationships established, or from the effects of age, maturity, and social relations changing their motivation to move along a spectrum from harm reduction to abstinence.

These principles subsequently influenced the UK Advisory Council on the Misuse of Drugs in its landmark recommendations to government. The Advisory Council report endorsed the harm reduction approach with its key message that 'the spread of HIV is a greater danger to individual and public health than drug misuse. Accordingly, services which aim to minimise HIV risk behaviour by all available means should take precedence in development plans' and that 'We must therefore be prepared to work with those who continue to misuse drugs to help them reduce the risks involved in doing so, above all the risk of acquiring or spreading HIV' (4).

Whilst these developments were taking place in Liverpool in the spring of 1986, it was a different story at the national level. I had enjoyed a close relationship with Chief Medical Officer Sir Donald Acheson since my Southampton days when he had been dean at the medical school. He had been particularly supportive behind the scenes when I had led a campaign against the construction of a private American hospital in the grounds of the teaching hospital there in the early 1980s and after my return to Liverpool I received occasional handwritten notes from him. He was aware of what we were doing with syringe exchange and in one of his notes he shared with me the frustrations he was experiencing in trying to convince prudish government ministers of the need for much greater frankness in engaging with the public on the delicate issues of risky sexual behaviour. Years later Norman Fowler, the Secretary of State for Health at the time, was to publish an account in which he would confront this issue and the delays in official response to the public health threat; in his view the blame lay elsewhere than in his own department!

Back in Liverpool the response to the new services from drug users was swift and impressive. A range of user-friendly and non-judgmental services, which were attractive to large numbers of drug users, were set up. This included substitute prescribing using methadone and did not exclude the provision of heroin itself and even heroin reefers. The imperative was to keep our patients away from impure street drugs and provide them with safer options. Outreach developed as a way to get in touch with those drug users not attracted to other services offering basic primary care interventions: information, advice, and clean injecting equipment.

That summer the news broke from Edinburgh, where the police had adopted a heavy-handed approach to drug users found with injecting equipment on their persons, that several dozen babies had been born who were HIV+. Drug injectors had taken to avoiding the prospects of arrest for possession of syringes by using drug dens instead where they would share syringes. Armed with this devastating data, Sir Donald Acheson was able to persuade Norman Fowler to allow him to establish a small number of pilots of syringe exchange. Having been under the radar since early in the year, and now with the experience of engagement with some hundreds of drug injectors who were moving towards safe injection, we put our hands up and became one of those pilots. Our studies were beginning to show that out of intravenous drug users seen at our services 85 per cent were likely not to have shared equipment in the previous month.

In the first 10 months, 733 drug users came to the syringe exchange in Maryland Street in the centre of Liverpool, appropriately in Hope Street between the Anglican and Roman Catholic cathedrals. By 1988 we had developed the scheme into a new type of primary care service for users, offering advice on safer injecting, treatment for abscesses, other injecting-related health problems, and HIV testing with hepatitis vaccination being offered later. Drug users were also attracted to the Drug Dependency Unit, which began to offer maintenance prescribing rather than just detoxification. By the late 1980s drug treatment services in Mersey were responsible for one-third of the methadone prescribed in England with syringe exchange schemes and drug treatment units being established throughout the region as the epidemic of drug use waxed.

Over the next five years many of the original objectives of our harm reduction approach were met. We made contact with about 50 per cent (10,000) of the high-risk drug-using population of Merseyside and considerably reduced the sharing of needles and syringes. Most drug users seeking treatment accepted oral substitute drugs with others offered injectables. The use of street drugs was reduced and an added bonus was a steady reduction in drug-related crime. Perhaps most importantly was the dramatic impact on the ratio of injecting addicts who were HIV+ (see Box 5.3).

It is now over 30 years since the twin threat of HIV and injecting drug use confronted us and made us dig deep for solutions. At the beginning of this period cannabis and glue sniffing had been the main concern but with heroin

Box 5.3 Ratio of injecting addicts to numbers who are HIV+ (1991)

South West Thames	18.8:1
Mersey	82.4:1
UK	4.3:1

came cocaine and an increasing range of substances including hallucinogenic 'dance' drugs and later designer drugs in ever-increasing variety. Poly-drug use became widespread. The initial societal response was to frame illicit drug use as criminal rather than medical issues with strong demographic divisions of attitude towards it depending on whether people had grown up with the phenomenon or were drawn into moral panic by tabloid headlines. Certainly serious health implications could be a consequence of the use of street drugs lacking the quality control of licensed pharmaceuticals. One example came in the year 2000 when an unusual increase in the morbidity and mortality of injecting drug users in the UK and Ireland was reported, including a number of deaths in the North West of England. Our involvement in the subsequent investigation led to collaboration with the regional police forces to secure forensic samples for laboratory analysis and the identification of a range of dangerous pathogens including *Clostridium botulinum* in the samples.

Whilst the adverse medical and health consequences of illicit drug taking could be clear enough, so too were the consequences of a massive trade being controlled by criminal gangs with its related violence and turf war murders. In addition thousands of young people's reputations and careers were damaged by casual association with recreational drug use and the prisons filled up with low-level drug dealers. As drug taking of all kinds moved from being epidemic to endemic the climate of public opinion began to shift in the general direction of harm reduction and the decriminalization of drug use towards a medical model as developed in Portugal.

Today there is clear indication that the millennial generation is not only using less drugs but is also beginning to turn away from the excessive alcohol consumption which had itself achieved epidemic proportions over the same period. When it comes to heroin the ebbing tide has begun to reveal an ageing cohort of injectors who are susceptible to drug-related death in association with generally poor health after years of abuse. The cause of death in these cases is often accidental overdose, something that could be remedied by the prompt administration of the antidote naloxone. In Liverpool between 2013 and 2016, sadly 109 drug users died from overdoses in this way. Ironically, the city that pioneered harm reduction in the 1980s has been one of the last to embrace a policy of ready availability of naloxone.

Turning the tide on alcohol abuse became a major focus of public health work from the 1980s onwards at national and local levels. Historically low price levels of alcoholic drinks combined with exotically flavoured novelty products to appeal to younger drinkers and a relaxation of licensing hours to regenerate the economic core of the industrial cities. The result was alcohol-fuelled chaos

Box 5.4 A cautionary tale: Teenager's stomach removed after drinking cocktail

Designer drugs and 'legal highs' were not the only exotic innovations to turn up as hazards to teenage life in the new millennium. On 4 October 2012 18-year-old Gaby Scanlon was out celebrating her birthday in Oscar's Wine Bar in Lancaster. She collapsed in agony after drinking her second Jagermeister cocktail containing liquid nitrogen. Her life was saved by removing her stomach in an emergency operation. The owners of the bar were subsequently fined £100,000.

in the night-time economy. In the North West one response was to develop Healthy Nightlife initiatives based on public health principles.

An important voice for public health over the past twenty years has undoubtedly been that of Sir Ian Gilmore, Liverpool gastroenterologist and former President of the Royal College of Physicians, who made the issue his own once he had started seeing relatively young patients in his clinics suffering from advanced liver disease. Sir Ian's significant contribution to public health illustrates the power of a respected senior clinical voice taking up a prominent position on a serious public health matter. The all-too-frequent schism between clinical practice and prevention has meant that the opportunity for others to contribute in this way is often missed. However, important examples are to be found over recent years that include Newcastle paediatrician Dr Hugh Jackson, who established the Child Accident Prevention Trust; London cardiologist Dr Keith Ball, who was one of the founders of the Coronary Prevention Group; and Cardiff surgeon Professor Jonathan Shepherd, whose work on shatterproof glasses in bars and clubs has led to important falls in the incidence of facial injury where these have been adopted. In Liverpool, venereologist and sexual health consultant Dr Peter Carey played a similarly important part as we got to grips with HIV/AIDS. (See box 5.4.)

HIV/AIDS

The advent of HIV and AIDS into the United Kingdom in the early 1980s was initially a slow burn. As elsewhere in the developed world there was initial inertia as a new disease that apparently affected only a stigmatized minority and was of little interest to mainstream clinicians and researchers, politicians, the media, the pharmaceutical industry, and the general public, failed to register on the urgent radar screen. It was only when this terrifying illness, which was apparently universally fatal, began to affect women and children as well as blood transfusion recipients, straight men, and drug injectors that those responsible for protecting the public health began to pay attention. Several years were lost, not least in Central and sub-Saharan Africa where the causal virus had probably been extracting a serious toll for some time before it reached Western countries. These events have been forensically described by Randy Shilts in his moving account *And The Band Played On*, by Peter Piot in *No Time To Lose*, and most recently by David France in his account *How to Survive a Plague*. In 2014, in a poignant replay of many of the same dynamics, there was a catastrophic failure of the global leaders of public health to respond to another deadly new virus, Ebola, which had seemingly emerged from the same part of Africa.

In Liverpool and the North West of England, our fortuitous encounter with Glen Margo together with the imaginative support we had enjoyed from chairman Sir Donald Wilson and, under the radar, Sir Donald Acheson in London had given us an opportunity to get on the front foot. Nevertheless it was not plain sailing. We were greatly helped in our efforts to move upstream of the virus by the dedicated involvement of local venereologist Dr Peter Carey, who had long worked in the Liverpool Seaman's Dispensary and the Royal Liverpool Hospital and who brought non-judgmental commitment, enthusiasm, and energy to bear in mobilizing a clinical response to prevention. Over the ensuing years we developed systematic programmes of education and intervention that built on the networks created in the days of the Liverpool Project and the beginnings of syringe exchange. The responsive services included extensive collaborative outreach especially with the gay community and commercial sex workers as the full picture of the epidemic unfolded. Through the work of the North West Public Health Observatory we were able to build a comprehensive picture of the people and places at most risk to inform targeted health education and clinical intervention. One spin-off of the work at this time with the widespread promotion of safe sexual practices was a reduction in the incidence of other sexually transmitted infections including gonorrhoea.

On Friday 21 November 1986, Norman (now Lord) Fowler, Secretary of State for Social Services, introduced a debate on AIDS in the House of Commons for the first time, over 5 years since the first report of its complications had appeared in the Morbidity and Mortality Weekly Report of the Centres for Disease Control in Atlanta on 5 June 1981. Sir Donald Acheson had been working away behind the scenes but it was too late for many who had already died from the disease. In his introductory remarks the minister said that 'No-one should underestimate how serious the threat is—in this country as in most of the rest of the world', before continuing: 'the disease is believed to be invariably fatal.

There is no cure, nor any immediate prospect of one. So it is a deadly threat. And already in this country there have been 565 cases of which 284 have died (5)' Some of the stigmatizing, judgmental, and prejudicial attitudes of the time were exposed in a further section of the speech: 'In the main, these are homosexuals or drug addicts or their partners. In addition there are the tragic cases of haemophiliacs who have been infected with contaminated blood and [hand written on my personal copy from Sir Donald Acheson of the minister's speech "worst of all"] of small babies who have been affected by their mothers' (5).

Norman Fowler continued to describe the proposed programme of public education measures which Sir Donald had finally managed to have adopted. On his visit to Liverpool to deliver the Duncan Lecture two years later, Sir Donald shared with us the public service material, including frank media messages about safe sex, that had been deployed to keep British servicemen free of disease during the Second World War. Forty years later it had been proving hard to repeat the exercise despite the Chief Medical Officer drawing it to the government's attention! The responses to this new threat were to include newspaper and poster campaigns, a youth campaign using magazines, radio, and cinema and early in the new year a leaflet drop to all 23 million households accompanied by television and radio advertising to maximize its effect. In addition a Health Education Council leaflet 'Don't Aid AIDS' would be sent to all 11,000 pharmacies in the country for the public to pick them up. The Health Education Council itself was to disappear and be replaced by a Special Health Authority with a clear line of accountability to ministers and to Parliament.

The minister's anxiety about the squeamish sensitivities of some of his more prudish colleagues continued to colour his approach: 'Clearly, however, the advertising will have to go into detail and will have to use language which is easy to understand. It may be that some will be offended. I regret that—but I have to say that I believe the greater danger is that the message does not get over' (5). Two weeks later, on 2nd December, Chief Medical Officer Sir Donald Acheson wrote to all doctors in the country with an update on the situation and detailing the measures that should now be taken. In his letter Sir Donald makes clear that in future the risk of infection from the HIV virus was no longer confined to small groups of people. In his 2014 retrospective book, *AIDS, Don't Die of Prejudice*, Norman Fowler is quite clear that Prime Minister Margaret Thatcher, together with some of her cabinet colleagues and advisers, was responsible for blocking the implementation of earlier advice from the Chief Medical Officer.

In anticipation of a thawing of official attitudes to public information Howard Seymour and I had been scouring the world for imaginative and effective examples and materials. We thought we had struck gold in Norway with some brilliant animation cartoons designed for television and cinema. They were simple, amusing, engaging and so, we predicted, would be effective in engaging the public and opening up discussion about safer sex. In one of the pieces there are four animation characters—A, I, D, and S making up the letters of AIDS. The 'I' represents a character as an erect penis making an approach to the 'A' representing a female in a reclining position. The 'A' resists the 'I's' advances with appropriate noises until a condom appears and ensheaths the 'I', at which point the scenario becomes much more chummy.

We obtained permission from the Norwegians to use their material with the intention of broadcasting it in the North West television region and approached the Independent Television Companies Association for clearance to broadcast it. The reply from John Jackson, the Head of Copy Clearance, to Howard Seymour on 25 November 1986 is depressing: 'After careful consideration, we are in no doubt that all three visual treatments would offend viewers to an unacceptable degree, even allowing for the seriousness of the AIDS situation, and that it would be wrong to transmit them' (6).

In January 1987 the Government's public education campaign began. To us it felt like a missed opportunity. With the whole country teed up for a groundbreaking initiative, what did it consist of? The campaign with a strapline of 'Don't Die of Ignorance' majored on two short television and cinema clips, one of an iceberg and one of a volcano proclaiming the scary message but giving no helpful advice other than to read the leaflet that would be put through your door. Having secured the nation's attention in the age of monopoly broadcasting the failure of follow-through was predictable. What proportion of leaflets put through the letter box are ever read rather than accumulating behind the door? Around the country it fell to public health and clinical workers to roll up their sleeves and engage with real community-level education with the general public and the special groups who were especially at risk.

The appearance of HIV in the 1980s was but one manifestation of the changes in sexual behaviour that had accompanied and followed on from the sexual revolution of the 1960s with greater personal and sexual freedoms. A range of other sexually transmitted infections had begun to climb in incidence in the following years. Of particular note was the occurrence of chlamydia, which was associated with secondary infertility in women and which was becoming endemic among sexually active younger people. A series of studies which I commissioned at this time on Merseyside found a prevalence in contraceptive and other gynaecological clinics of around 10 per cent. This led to pilots of screening for the agent and in due course to a national screening programme. Gonorrhoea and syphilis, both diseases which we believed to have been consigned to history with the use of penicillin, also made a comeback during the 1980s and 1990s.

An outbreak of penicillin-resistant gonorrhoea among the clients of massage parlours and later a return of syphilis among HIV+ gay men who were seeking out other HIV+ men for unprotected sex, both in Greater Manchester, were examples of the incidents we had to handle into the 1990s. By this time our Heath Protection Team had developed a routine for such events, which required a multiagency and partnership response of declaring major public health incidents, chaired by myself as Director of Public Health. Faced with the massage parlour outbreak my first response was to request a list of the establishments concerned, much as you might with food establishments in an outbreak of food poisoning or contamination. That no such list existed reinforced my belief that that the registration and proper management of premises used for commercial sex along the lines that had long existed in the Netherlands was long overdue.

Problems worthy of attack—infectious diseases

'Problems worthy of attack prove their worth by hitting back.'

—Piet Hein

The belief that the advent of modern medicines together with immunization and vaccination was leading to the demise of infectious disease was in part behind the rundown of public health in the immediate post-war period. In the United Kingdom the abolition of the post of local Medical Officer of Health in 1974 and the creation of a new position, that of Community Physician, within health authorities had been indicative of the mindset which saw the public health of the future as being primarily about the planning of health services. That these new arrangements only lasted 14 years was because it soon became apparent that the neglect of traditional public health concerns in the form of infectious disease within the community would have political as well as health consequences. Sir Donald Acheson's enquiry, *Public Health in England*, in 1988 came about as the result of serious failings in infectious disease control that had led to a salmonella outbreak at the Stanley Royd psychogeriatric hospital in Wakefield in which 19 patients died together with a second serious public health failure at Stafford hospital involving Legionnaires' disease. In Stafford the outbreak, which was associated with the hospital air conditioning system, led to 68 confirmed cases with 22 deaths, a case fatality rate of just over 30 per cent. The upshot included the establishment of new Control of Communicable Disease posts that linked the NHS to local authorities where the post holder was to be an adviser.

Salmonella was to become something of a theme in 1988 with a highly publicized incident involving Health Minister Edwina Currie, who had a propensity for attracting media headlines, and a major epidemic of contamination of eggs from poultry with the organism *Salmonella*. Throughout the 1980s cases of food poisoning by *Salmonella enteritidis* had been steadily increasing, usually associated with contamination of hens' eggs, frequently when used in uncooked or lightly cooked forms. In November 1988 it became newsworthy when the Department of Health in London reported that there had recently been 26 confirmed outbreaks and that there could be many more. Speaking on radio in London on 23rd November, Sir Donald Acheson sought to put over a measured assessment of the situation, steering a path between imparting public information and alarm. Putting matters in perspective he summarized that 'bearing in mind that 30 million eggs are eaten every day, the proportion of infected eggs is a very small proportion indeed' (7). He went on to give down-to-earth practical advice about the use of raw eggs whilst infected flocks could be traced and the infection eradicated. Two weeks later on 3rd December junior Minister of Health Edwina Currie weighed in with the claim on television that 'most of the egg production in this country, sadly, is now affected with salmonella' (8). Her remarks caused outrage with poultry farmers and egg sales fell by 60 per cent with the slaughter of 4 million hens and she was forced to resign before Christmas. The importance of this episode is in the way it crystallizes the delicacy of the relationship between the technical and the political in questions of public health. Evidence-based advice is essential to good government and the protection of public health. A wise politician will know when it is appropriate to front-up matters of public concern and when to let the shoulders of their professional advisers take the strain. The public is unforgiving if amateurs get it wrong.

The 1988 Acheson report was a wake-up call that the infectious diseases remained core business for public health. Bovine spongeiform encephalitis (BSE or mad cow disease) had made an appearance in 1986, to be followed by Hong Kong bird flu in 1997, SARS in 2003, swine flu in 2009, and Ebola in 2014. An outbreak of plague in India in 1994 led to panic measures internationally, hospital- and community-acquired antibiotic-resistant infection (HAI) became a regular concern, and following the terrorist attack on the World Trade Centre in New York in 2001, bio-terrorism and the threat of 'white powder' anthrax incidents led to a renewed focus on biological threats to public health. At the local level, also in 2001, a massive outbreak of foot-and-mouth disease in cattle, not least in Cumbria, led to tens of thousands of cattle being slaughtered and burned in medieval funeral pyres with devastating agricultural and health impact on both farmers and country dwellers that would bring with it a long tail. In 2002 in Barrow-in-Furness the third largest reported outbreak of *Legionella* would challenge the clinical system of a small community but it would rise to the task. (See Box 5.5.)

Box 5.5 Some infectious disease threats to public health from 1986

Bovine spongeiform encephalitis, 1986–
Salmonella in eggs, 1988
Plague, 1994
Bird flu (Hong Kong) 1997
Foot-and-mouth disease, 2001
Legionella, 2002
SARS, 2003
H1N1 swine flu, 2009
Ebola, 2014

Bovine spongeiform encephalitis, 1986

Concern over food hygiene and contamination goes back to biblical times. Former Chief Environmental Health Officer Mike Eastwood was fond of quoting the Old Testament book of Leviticus to the effect that it was not allowed to eat fallen stock but was acceptable to sell it to the next village. In the case of BSE the origins of this disease, caused by pathogenic proteins called prions, arose as a result of animal carcasses being recycled to livestock in animal feed-stuffs in defiance of the precautionary principle.

The first cases of this irreversible and devastating disease, which became known as new variant Creutzfeldt–Jakob disease or nvCJD when it affected humans, occurred in 1986 and came to political attention in 1987. It is characterized by progressive neurological deterioration, dementia, personality changes, and ultimately death. In May 1990, in a state of uncertainty about the disease's origin and being apparently more concerned about its economic impact on the agricultural industry than its impact on public health, the minister responsible for food safety in England at the time, John Gummer, chose to reassure the public by feeding a beef burger to his daughter Cornelia in a press conference. His daughter's friend was one of those who subsequently died from the disease. By the time the causal relationships involving the food chain, the prion, and the illness had been pinned down and stringent control measures introduced later in the 1990s, thousands of people had been affected with many deaths. The subsequent Phillips enquiry into the Government's handling of the crisis was critical of aspects of the risk management and communication and of the delays in intervening. In particular it felt that the possibility of a risk to humans as well as to animals was not communicated to the public or to those whose job was to implement and enforce the precautionary principle.

One lesson of this affair for public health advisers to policy makers is the importance of an audit trail of advice in order that the allocation of decision-making responsibility can be properly allocated in the event of flawed policy and action. The minister involved, John Gummer, was subsequently promoted to the House of Lords.

Avian flu, SARS, and swine flu, a triple whammy? And then Ebola!

The great pandemic of influenza that swept the world in 1919 came in the aftermath of the First World War. With a European population weakened by years of conflict, environmental degradation, and poor nutrition, a new virus introduced from North America by troops arriving to join the battle was able to take root and sweep through the continent and beyond. Apparently originating in an army camp in Kansas the influenza reached Europe in the winter of 1918 and is estimated to have killed over 100 million people worldwide. Subsequently it transpired that survivors of the pandemic appeared to be over-represented in clusters of Parkinson's disease which could not be accounted for by any other explanation.

The nature of the influenza virus with frequent changes in its structure has proved a challenge to clinical researchers searching for effective vaccines. Global outbreaks emerge annually, usually in the winter months, involving different strains of the virus, with deaths mostly in the young, older people, and those with pre-existing health problems. Pandemics comparable to the 1919 outbreak, which came to be known as Spanish influenza, seem to occur every 20–30 years with more than a million deaths in each of the 1958 ('Asian flu') and 1968 ('Hong Kong flu') outbreaks. One of the worrying aspects of the virus is its propensity to evolve into new pathogenic forms in domestic animals that live in close proximity to humans such as pigs, horses, and poultry, where zoonotic cross-infection becomes a possibility. The speed of modern global transport has raised the spectre of pandemics today being able to spread much more rapidly than in the past. It is against this background that the two most recent global outbreaks together with the outbreak of severe acute respiratory syndrome in November 2002 should be viewed.

Hong Kong bird flu, 1997

The outbreak of Hong Kong bird flu began in May 1997 with a health worker who had become infected with the H5N1 virus after contact with a boy who had died having apparently contracted the disease from contact with chickens. By

December health officials reported that 30 people had been infected and that there had been four deaths but believed that the transmission was from bird to man rather than making the leap to human-to-human transmission.

With a daily import of 75,000 chickens from mainland China into one of the most densely populated urban spaces in the world it put Hong Kong's Director of Public Health (later to become Director General of the World Health Organization), Margaret Chan, in a difficult position. With the eyes of the world on her she convened a Sunday evening meeting at which the decision was taken to slaughter Hong Kong's entire poultry flock, having already stopped all poultry imports. The cull covered 160 chicken farms, 39 mixed poultry farms, and two wholesale markets. The total number of birds killed amounted to 1.25 million and the compensation bill reached £5 million.

Shortly afterwards I was visiting Hong Kong to support Margaret Chan's predecessor Dr S. H. Lee in launching WHO's Healthy Cities initiatives across the city. S. H. was renowned for his political wisdom and skill at implementing public health interventions in a complex environment. His analysis of the root cause of the outbreak focused on the wet markets for fish and poultry to be found in every neighbourhood and where environmental health standards were often poor or non-existent. On the basis of 'never wasting a good crisis' S. H. had decided that now was the opportunity to convince the Hong Kong Government of the need for a new initiative on environmental health. Together we did the circuit of all government departments where productive conversations with civil servants and politicians had the desired result (see Figure 5.1).

Severe acute respiratory syndrome (SARS), 2002–3

SARS is a viral respiratory disease of zoonotic origin caused by a corona virus. It produces flu-like respiratory symptoms and can lead rapidly to death from pneumonia. Between November 2002 and July 2003, an outbreak of SARS in southern China caused almost 800 deaths from 8000 cases in 37 countries, a case fatality rate of almost 10 per cent. The epidemic appears to have started in the Guangdong province in November 2002 but Chinese officials failed to inform the World Health Organization of the outbreak until February 2003, resulting in the slowness of the international response and a later apology from China. Coincidentally, I was again visiting China at the end of 2002 and came across a small circulation English language newspaper in my Beijing hotel which carried a report of the early cases. Recognizing that this might be of importance I faxed it to colleagues back in the UK for their information. It was only when the row blew up about the failure of notification by the Chinese that I discovered that the fax had never got further than the fax machine in England!

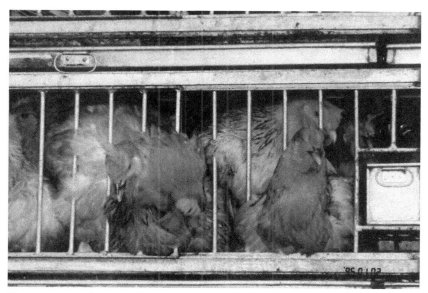

Figure 5.1 Typical scene in a Hong Kong wet market for poultry.
Reproduced courtesy of John Ashton.

Pandemic H1N1 influenza (swine flu), 2009

The pandemic of influenza of 2009 originated in pigs in central Mexico and led to more than 17,000 deaths worldwide. After the avian flu of 1997 and SARS in 2003, the public health world, the mass media, and the population generally had been sensitized to the idea that a pandemic might be on the way. The first cases were identified in April 2009, leading to the closure of public places in Mexico City in an attempt to contain the virus which seemed to have emerged from a combination of bird, swine, and human flu viruses. Once person-to-person cases had appeared and inter-country spread was a reality, Margaret Chan, who was now Director General of the World Health Organization, declared a global public health emergency, the WHO's first ever.

The first cases in the United Kingdom occurred towards the end of the month, a number of them being in schoolchildren from private schools who had been on long-haul school trips to Mexico, among these being cases among children from a school in Cumbria. Our early efforts at ring containment of cases by traditional public health measures of isolation and hygiene backed up by anti-viral drugs were aborted at the end of June. At this point the Chief Medical Officer, Sir Liam Donaldson, decided that with extensive community-level spread across the south-east of England and into the Midlands, ring containment was no longer practical, that in future anti-viral drugs would only be given to people showing symptoms and that the tracing of contacts would stop. The shift to a treatment as opposed to a containment approach was announced on 2nd July.

The pandemic tailed off after November 2009 with WHO declaring the outbreak over on 10 August 2010. At this point the recriminations began, with critics claiming that WHO had exaggerated the danger and allegations that major pharmaceutical companies had organized a campaign of panic to sell anti-viral agents. WHO's response was that it had adhered to explicit virological and epidemiological criteria in taking the steps it had done. In situations such as this, public health is caught between a rock and a hard place, the need to make the impact of prevention and intervention visible being urgent if at all possible. The price of failing to protect the public's health is condemnation. Margaret Chan's experience with bird flu in Hong Kong was presumably important in her decision. The impact of this latest challenge on the later Ebola outbreak in West Africa would be difficult to call.

Ebola, 2014

Many of the issues that had surfaced with other major outbreaks of infectious disease over the previous 30 years surfaced again when Ebola appeared in West Africa in the spring of 2014. Here was a new exotic virus of zoonotic origin, affecting some of the poorest people in the world with poorly developed medical services. Despite the virus having been identified at about the same time as HIV and against a similar backdrop, there had been no real effort to research it for preventive vaccines or treatment and the environmental and development issues that underpinned the susceptibility of the local populations of West Africa to its ravages had gone unaddressed. The international community was caught flat-footed and WHO itself failed to act in a timely manner, perhaps chastened by the criticism that had followed the swine flu 5 years earlier. It was only when cases began to appear in citizens of developed countries that the alert was taken up and even then a biological narrowness of thinking restricted the range of interventions. It was to take the involvement of anthropologists providing insights into the influences on risky traditional burial practices before effective action began. To make matters worse the failure to frame those most at risk as the health care workers and those involved in burial led to resources being spread too thin. This became relevant, not least in the approach to screening travellers returning to the United Kingdom from West Africa where a failure to concentrate the screening on returning health care workers led to the nurse Pauline Cafferkey going undiagnosed at Heathrow airport, and then being blamed for her own condition on her return from an admirable humanitarian mission.

Legionella

Legionnaires' disease, caused by the *Legionella* bacterium, is so called because it was first identified in an outbreak among delegates to an American Legion conference in Philadelphia in 1976 with 28 deaths. Characterized by a flu-like illness leading to atypical pneumonia, it is usually caused by contamination of hot water tanks, cooling towers, and institutional air conditioning units that have not been properly maintained. Infection is not spread from person to person, the incubation period is usually 2–10 days, and the mortality rate is typically between 10 and 30 per cent.

An outbreak in Barrow-in-Furness occurred in July and August of 2002 and was associated with an air conditioning unit at a local authority arts and leisure centre. Members of the general public were exposed to the organism as they walked through a passageway adjacent to the building where it subsequently transpired that there had been a failure of plant maintenance. Following reports of a significant increase in admissions to the local hospital with atypical pneumonia the first case was identified on 30th July and confirmed the following day. When the second case was confirmed on Friday 2nd August I decided to treat this as a major public health incident and convened an outbreak control meeting. This was occurring almost a year after the terrorist attack on the World Trade Centre in New York, which had led to the creation of the Health Protection Agency in England, bringing together the biological, chemical, and radiological and contingency planning aspects of health protection. It would be a test not only of these new national arrangements but also of the local arrangements which we had put previously in place.

At the national level the new Health Protection Agency had brought together the Public Health Laboratory Service, the National Radiological Protection Board, the Centre for Applied Microbiological Research, and the National Focus for Chemical Incidents. Established as a Special Health Authority in response to the threat to public security posed by international terrorism, to public health workers on the ground it felt like yet one more in a constant stream of structural reorganizations imposed on the National Health Service by politicians insensitive to the disruption to interagency working and organizational memory. At the local level we felt we had already achieved what was functionally necessary without structural change but believed that whatever the national level threw at us we would respond to the best of our ability. In the case of a major public health incident involving *Legionella*, this meant bringing together the key players round the table (see Box 5.6).

This episode coincided with the spectacle of the Commonwealth Games in Manchester, where I was committed as one of the medical commissioners,

Box 5.6 Members of the Barrow-in-Furness incident group

- Public health—NHS North West Regional Director of Public Health, local directors of Public Health and Consultants in Communicable Disease Control.
- Environmental health—Barrow Borough Council Head of Environmental Health
- Microbiology—Morecambe Bay Acute Hospitals NHS Trust consultant microbiologists and North West Regional Microbiology Director
- Intelligence—NHS North West Intelligence Managers
- Communications—Morecambe Bay Acute Hospitals NHS Trust Communications Manager and NHS North West Communications Manager
- Health and Safety Executive

tasked with overseeing the drug testing of the world's leading athletes. With the Outbreak Control Room being set up in Barrow, 100 miles from the Commonwealth Stadium in Manchester, it was a question of juggling Commonwealth Games on-duty shifts with commutes up the M6 motorway until the local Public Health Director, the very hands-on Nick Gent, was able to break his family holiday and fly home. The number of cases rose steadily and was to reach a final tally of 179, the third largest outbreak in the world literature. (The largest was 449 cases in Murcia, in Spain in 2003.)

Despite the organizational disruption imposed from above, the local multi-agency response kicked in like a well-oiled machine. With the benefit of high-quality family doctors and a small but committed local hospital laboratory and clinical staff, cases were swiftly identified and started on treatment, whilst the environmental measures needed to deal with the source of the problem were rapidly put in place. With Nick Gent back in the local driving seat, I was able to report to Prime Minister Tony Blair at the closing ceremony of the games on Sunday 4th August that the outbreak was under control. The final death toll being 7, a case fatality rate of less than 4 per cent.

What the Barrow *Legionella* outbreak demonstrated was that strong local public health arrangements with good interagency whole system relationships can respond quickly and effectively to even quite exotic public health emergencies. As so often in such events, the national level seems remote and by the time it becomes involved the incident may well have acquired its own momentum. Such resilience appears to have been missing in Stafford almost 20 years before where the case fatality rate was many times as great. In Barrow, the subsequent prosecutions of the local authority revealed that a maintenance contract on the air conditioning system that was incriminated had been cancelled as a means to save money.

Measles, mumps, and rubella (MMR): The special case of complacency and the need for vigilance

As a child growing up in post Second World War Liverpool, I experienced many of the potentially serious, common childhood infections along with my siblings and schoolmates. In those days before the availability of the universal vaccination programmes that later became available I contracted measles, German measles (rubella), whooping cough (pertussis), chicken pox (varicella), and mumps (parotitis), and spent 6 weeks in the Alder Hey Children's Hospital with suspected meningitis. Although deaths from a number of these diseases had become greatly reduced in previous years on account of improved nutrition and the improved availability of medical care, cases were still occurring together with tuberculosis and periodic outbreaks of diphtheria and paralytic polio. Vaccinations against diphtheria, pertussis, tuberculosis, and polio were provided to all children by 1956 and subsequently against an increasing range of other pathogens.

Before the introduction of measles vaccine, notifications of measles varied between 60,000 and 800,000 cases a year with biennial peaks once the number of susceptible newborns in the community had reached levels sufficient for outbreaks to take root. After the introduction of measles vaccine initial coverage remained low with annual notifications of between 50,000 and 100,000 and an average of 13 measles deaths each year. The introduction of the measles, mumps, and rubella (MMR) vaccine in 1988 was a game-changer, enabling protection to be offered not only against measles but also these two other potentially serious infections with their potential for complications that included inflammation of the testes, meningitis, and deafness (mumps), and a range of problems, in particular the congenital rubella syndrome with cataracts, deafness, and heart and brain complications born to the infants of pregnant mothers who had been infected (rubella). By combining the three vaccines it was possible to simplify the increasing vaccination schedule for young children with the objective of securing a 95 per cent coverage rate, to secure so-called 'herd' immunity, which would prevent outbreaks of any of these three infections. By the late 1990s most regions of England, including the North West, were able to claim in excess of

90 per cent child population vaccination with MMR and be well on the way to a historic public health goal.

On 28 February 1998, British gastroenterologist and researcher Andrew Wakefield published a paper with 12 other authors in *The Lancet* which claimed to have identified a new syndrome in which there was a link between MMR vaccination and childhood autism. Although the research was subsequently discredited and Wakefield struck off the UK medical register for publishing fraudulent research, the impact of the widely reported *Lancet* paper was dramatic with falls in uptake of the triple vaccine which were as low as 70 per cent in more affluent areas of London and the South East.

There followed a 10-year struggle to retrieve the situation which was characterized by a protracted and acrimonious dispute between, often middle class, opponents of the vaccine and a clinical and science community that had been caught off-guard and was often uncomfortable engaging in full-out media advocacy. It fell to public health directors to front up the arguments on radio, television, and the print media and to ensure that frontline health workers themselves had not been taken in by the negative publicity. This could be particularly difficult when it came to handling the arguments of families who genuinely believed they had a child who had experienced vaccine damage. It was not helped by a cultural context in which half the population of the country had studied no science after the age of 16 years and in which many mainstream media insisted on giving equal air time to opponents of MMR as well as to the clinical and scientific community with its evidence base as to vaccine safety. In bringing the North West coverage back up above 90 per cent within five years my wife and I took the decision that on this occasion it was appropriate to make public the vaccination of our own young son. This was in contrast with Prime Minister Blair's reluctance to comment on the vaccination status of his youngest child, leading to public opprobrium, whilst some opponents of the vaccine sought to compare our action with that of the government minister who had publicly appeared to feed his daughter on beef burger at the height of the BSE crisis.

Protecting public health in emergencies—thinking the unthinkable and doing the essential

The threats to life from the natural and built environments vary enormously around the world. Those of us fortunate enough to live in geologically stable places with moderate weather systems and functioning democracies may take for granted what others can only dream of. The prevention of environmental disasters in urban and rural areas is dependent on robust systems of precaution and awareness at home, in the workplace, at leisure, and as we move between the settings of everyday life. The price of security is vigilance, anticipation, and resilience across whole systems, large and small. Usually when things go wrong they are the result of a convergence of factors, any one of which might have led to a near miss but cumulatively creates a sense of the inevitable. The outcome can be a devastating loss of life, serious injury, and longstanding detriment to mental health. Sensible societies plan for the unthinkable and do their best to avoid it. If the worst should happen they are likely to be prepared to minimize the consequences. In the late 1980s a succession of disasters grabbed the news headlines, beginning with the sinking of the *Herald of Free Enterprise* ferry boat off the Belgium coast on 6 March 1987 with the loss of 193 lives, followed soon after by a fire at Kings Cross Station in London that killed 31 on November 18th of the same year. On July 6th of the following year 167 workers were to perish in an explosion and fire on board the Alpha Piper oil rig in the North Sea. These should have been a wake-up call for civil defence against large-scale emergencies.

The Hillsborough Stadium football disaster

My personal baptism of fire began on a beautiful spring morning in April 1989 when I set off from Liverpool with two of my sons and a nephew to attend the semi-final football match between Liverpool and Nottingham Forest at the Hillsborough Stadium in Sheffield. Within a few hours 95 supporters would be dead with a further death sometime later, thousands of people's lives would be changed forever and the reputations of senior figures in the public and emergency services damaged beyond redemption. It would take almost 30 years for the subsequent cover-up of responsibilities to be fully exposed, too late in many cases for proper lessons to be learnt and healing to take place.

As an academic public health physician at that time I had no direct responsibility for emergency planning or response. However, as a spectator, doctor, and citizen finding himself in the middle of a disaster on the football terraces it fell to me to implement a system of triage close to the scene.

The disaster occurred as a result of a sequence of decisions and events that cascaded into tragedy. The football ground was tired and unsuitable for such a major game, the terracing for standing supporters behind the Leppings Lane goal having been caged in to prevent spectator pitch invasions; crush barriers designed to keep closely packed supporters safe had been removed; the larger following of Liverpool supporters had been allocated the smaller of the two end terraces; an inexperienced senior police officer who had been put in charge of the game failed to implement proper procedures for marshalling spectators and panicked when things went wrong. He then initiated a cover-up in which the supporters were blamed for events outside their control. The tragedy happened when large numbers of fans were directed through an underground tunnel that was far too small to accommodate them safely and many were crushed to death within the confines of a caged pen, unable to escape whilst police officers assuming crowd trouble refused an escape route through gates onto the pitch in front. My involvement in the area immediately behind the tunnel was to coordinate the first response in the absence of any leadership from the emergency services, to triage and despatch the injured to hospital, and to certify death among the casualties. It became clear over the course of the acute phase that not only had there been a disaster of terrible proportions but also a catastrophic failure to coordinate a multiagency emergency response. In the meantime, I would be moving from my academic base in the University of Liverpool to take up the new role as Regional Director of Public Health. Once the implications of this became clear, that I would have a direct input and responsibility with health emergency planning, I was determined that the North West would never be caught out the way South Yorkshire had on 15 April 1989.

At the time of my moving to the regional health authority in 1993, the world of emergency and contingency planning was in a state of flux. Although the Cold War had ended with the collapse of the Soviet Union in December 1991, the first Gulf War between Western powers and the forces of Iraq's Saddam Hussain had recently taken place, and the Irish Republican Army (IRA) was still a threat to civilian and civic targets in the United Kingdom. The Good Friday Agreement that would bring the beginnings of peace in Northern Ireland was still 5 years away (10 April 1998) and it would be 8 years before the terrorist attacks on the World Trade Centre in New York would usher in a new era of insecurity leading to new challenges for health protection. By September 1993, Tom Hobday had long since left his position as head of Defence Medical Planning at the regional health authority and the plethora of Cold War Emergency Rest Centre Plans had disappeared from the walls of his old office. Nevertheless, the approach to health emergency planning was still by an emphasis on Cold War secrecy; it was a million miles from the community resilience building that I had witnessed on travels to New Zealand and North America where natural disasters were not uncommon and active citizenship was the norm. My experience at Hillsborough had convinced me that there must be another way, one that was much more suited to a modern public health that stressed partnership and public engagement. I would have plenty of opportunity to test this belief over the next 13 years as a succession of major incidents came along in the North West region and later in Cumbria. (See Box 5.7.)

These could be described as either being of an environmental 'accidental' nature or involving some measure of intent through social disorder or violence.

Box 5.7 Major incidents in the North West and Cumbria, 1993–2006

1. Environmental emergencies
   - Morecambe Bay Cockler Drownings, 5 February 2004
   - Cumbria floods, 2005, 2009
   - Grayrigg train crash, 23 February 2007
   - Keswick school bus crash, 24 May 2010
2. Civil disorder/violence
   - IRA bomb attacks, Warrington, 26 February and 20 March 1993; Manchester, 15 June 1996
   - Aintree Racecourse, bomb threat evacuation, 5 April 1997
   - Kosovo refugee emergency, March–June 1999
   - National fuel dispute, 8–14 September 2000
   - West Cumbria mass shootings, 2 June 2010

Following the events of September 11th in America, attention became much more focused on the importance of proper preparedness. Around the country health emergency planning became a mainstream activity for the National Health Service and for public health directorates with an emphasis on training, desk top exercises, and full-scale emergency gaming. Comprehensive sets of action cards were produced which made explicit the responsibilities of individuals (see Box 5.8). In the British context it is normal for the chief police officer to convene and chair the Strategic Gold Command response to a major incident although other top-level partners can declare a major incident if appropriate. In the aftermath of the terrorist attacks in the USA on 11 September 2001, and subsequent anthrax and 'white powder' incidents, the arrangements were amended to put the director of public health in the chair in the event of a chemical or biological incident. The division of responsibilities into Strategic Gold Command together with Silver and Bronze as the implementation arm for action has endured for the best part of a hundred years.

Three terrorist threats—lessons from the IRA

In the space of four years the North West was affected by IRA-related incidents on three occasions. In 1993, on two occasions, bombs were detonated in

Box 5.8 Action card—director of public health (the first hour)

The primary role of the director of public health or deputy, in the event of a major incident, is to provide public health advice and to take a strategic overview of health needs.

On receipt of incident alert:

- ◆ Complete incident response form to record incident details.
- ◆ Start incident log to record all actions and decisions.
- ◆ Contact chief executive to inform of incident (confirm that NHS Strategic Health Commander has been alerted).

Incident update:

- ◆ Contact NHS Strategic Health Commander to obtain detailed understanding of the problem and potential impact.
- ◆ Assess scale and type of incident and public health response required.
- ◆ Decide on specific or urgent actions required.
- ◆ Confirm what public warning messages have been issued by police.

Contact national public health agency:

- ◆ In the event that the incident is chemical, biological, radiological, or nuclear, confirm that relevant section has been contacted.

Contact Regional Director of Public Health:

- ◆ Advise appropriate regional director(s) of public health.

Strategic Coordination Group (Gold Command):

- ◆ If Gold Command called, attend Major Incident Multiagency Teleconference or Gold Command meeting in Command Headquarters.

Scientific and technical advice cell (in the event of a chemical, biological, radiological, or nuclear incident):

- ◆ At the request of the police and in discussion with the National Public Health agency, set up a scientific and technical advice cell (STAC).
- ◆ Make the decision as to who will chair the STAC.
- ◆ If the incident crosses county or country border, public health director will become the cross-border link.

Warrington. On the second occasion three-year-old Jonathan Ball and twelve-year-old Tim Parry were killed and many people injured. The modus operandi of the IRA was to detonate two bombs within minutes of each other in order to catch first responders in the second blast; this was not known by the public and was a symptom of an approach to anti-terrorist planning which did not share information outside a close circle of professionals on a 'need to know basis'.

On the second occasion in June 1996, the IRA demonstrated greater ambition with an attempt to blow up the Arndale shopping centre in central Manchester. The explosion occurred at 10am, 17 minutes after a telephone warning had been received and the police had begun to evacuate 80,000 people from central Manchester. With the potential for mass casualties it was important that the National Health Service should be able to respond adequately; however, apart from a few medical accident and emergency consultants who were involved in drawing up a mass casualty plan, there had been little prior engagement of NHS or Department of Health staff. On hearing of the explosions I alerted members of the public health team and tried to contact the headquarters of the Department of Health in London. Not only was the HQ of the Manchester Health Authority closed and locked but the porter on the desk in London had no instructions as to what to do (it was a weekend!). This was hardly an indication of an organization ready to respond to an emergency either at the local or national levels. In the event large numbers of clinical staff went spontaneously to their places of work to volunteer for action. Fortunately they were not needed as there were so few casualties. This experience galvanized me on a mission to ensure that in future there would be full and proper engagement with health emergency planning of all parts of the NHS, managers as well as clinicians. As my own knowledge developed I made sure that public health teams had proper training and took my own team on a residential training course at the National Emergency Planning College; this included training the administrative and clerical staff as potential loggists in a large-scale disaster, able to maintain a minute-by-minute record of discussions held, decisions made, and actions taken, a record which has subsequent force as a legal and forensic document.

Following the Manchester bomb, progress was made in engaging with clinicians and managers but the involvement of community health workers and family doctors was elusive until the third IRA incident the following year. This incident at the world famous Grand National horse-racing steeplechase in Liverpool took the form of a bomb warning that transpired to be a hoax. On a cold, wet spring day in April 60,000 people from around the country and the world were stranded without adequate clothing or prescription medicines, while the police Gold Command concentrated on the supposed terrorist threat. By the time Dave Ward, my health emergency planning officer, insisted that a public health emergency be declared, night was closing in. Thousands of people had to be accommodated overnight and fed in schools and church halls around the city, family doctors and pharmacists had to be mobilized, and a response implemented that was as much social as medical but one in which the relevance of primary care was obvious. Invoking the spirit of the Second World War Blitz, the Liverpool people responded to the occasion to care for the strangers in their midst.

The collapse of former Yugoslavia—humanitarian repercussions for one region

From the end of the Second World War peace in Europe had lasted for the best part of 50 years until the civil war in Yugoslavia. The maintenance of peace had been made possible by the determination of the generation that had witnessed the horrors of war and by the subsequent institution building, leading to the creation of the European Union. However, the collapse of the Soviet Union in 1991 had created new uncertainties and opened up new fracture lines, not least those in the Balkans.

As city medical officer for Zagreb in Croatia, Slobodan Lang was close to the events as they unfolded. A profoundly humanitarian public health doctor, Slobodan had personal reasons for being sensitive to the irrational hostilities that arise because of cultural and religious differences; his paternal grandfather was president of the Jewish community of Vonkovci and he and his wife were killed during the Holocaust. Until the collapse of the Soviet Union, only a strong man in the form of Josep Broz Tito could hold the complex mixture of races and religions together that makes up the Balkan region with its historic enmities. With Tito's death in 1980, it all began to unravel.

By 1990, civil war was on the horizon and Slobodan could read the runes. That September, at the WHO Healthy Cities conference in Stockholm, he and I drafted a statement for delegates which identified the important spiritual prerequisites to health and the threat of hatred to public health (see Box 5.9).

This was a timely reminder as the Balkans slid into civil war that hatred and armed conflict were once again becoming among the greatest dangers to health and wellbeing. We needed to be reminded of the dreadful history of warfare and its impact on public health. In the seventeenth century military deaths accounted for 19 out of each million deaths, but by the twentieth century this had risen to 183. Furthermore whereas in the First World War civilians had accounted for only 10 per cent of deaths, in the most recent conflicts this had risen to 75 per cent and the Balkans would follow this pattern, accompanied by mass displacement of populations and the threat of the classical public health

Box 5.9 Tolerance and reconciliation, the spiritual prerequisites to health

'Hate is the biggest danger to health and the quality of life. Health workers and health services of all countries and in all communities have the responsibility to inform people about the health consequences of hate and to stimulate them to tolerance and reconciliation—reconciliation is also needed between people and the natural environment to which they owe their sustenance.

'Hate is the most dangerous inner pollution; it is the pollution of the spirit...

'Tolerance is not just the absence of hate. Tolerance is a positive inner, spiritual feeling of security, a desire and willingness to live in peace with all people. Freedom, democracy, human rights, respect, justice, solidarity and reconciliation are the tools evaluating our social relations, inner spirit and consciousness. They are mutually dependent and supportive. Nowhere can tolerance be developed for all times. Everybody should develop, promote, practice, cherish and sustain tolerance. Tolerance includes respect and support for all in freely choosing and living their own way of life. Tolerance also includes cooperation among groups and nations based on the principles of equity, solidarity and respect for all.' *Slobodan Lang/John Ashton, Stockholm, 24 September 1990*

consequences of starvation, squalor, epidemics, psychological trauma, and further cycles of violence.

The Stockholm statement was adopted by the Healthy Cities conference and was relayed from it to a number of parliaments by politician delegates, not least in the Baltic States were anxiety was growing about neighbouring political tensions. As the tragic events continued to unfold with primitive bloodletting and the rise of ethnic cleansing, many thousands of lives were lost. Slobodan continued to provide humanitarian leadership throughout the crisis as a mediator and negotiator, locally and internationally with the agencies of the United Nations. The emergency was to last a further 10 years, culminating with the Serbian invasion of Kosovo and a further humanitarian disaster.

The Kosovo Emergency

The struggle of Kosovo Muslims for greater independence within the Christian and Serb- dominated post-Tito Yugoslavia culminated in armed conflict lasting from 5 March 1998 until 11 June 1999. The fighting between the Kosovo Liberation Army (KLA), and the Yugoslav authorities, including Serb para-militaries, led to thousands of atrocities and deaths and the mass expulsion of Kosovar Albanians over the border into Macedonia. Later the United Nations Supreme Court was to find that there had been 'a systematic campaign of terror, including murders, rapes, arsons and severe maltreatment' (9) (of the Kosovo Albanians).

The humanitarian crisis reached a peak in the late spring of 1999 with over 100,000 refugees being accommodated in camps on the Macedonian side of the border with Kosovo (see Figure 5.2), and the involvement of NATO forces interceding on behalf of the besieged and displaced Kosovans. The United Kingdom became involved with other allied countries in responding to civilian distress and in arranging the evacuation of refugees who could not obtain medical care locally as local health services were overwhelmed. At this point a call for public health involvement met a response from Public Health Director Celia Duff, who began the process of prioritizing refugees for evacuation from the refugee camps. When it became apparent that the largest numbers were bound for the North West, first Nick Gent, later myself, continued the work that Celia had begun. By the beginning of June tens of thousands of men, women, and

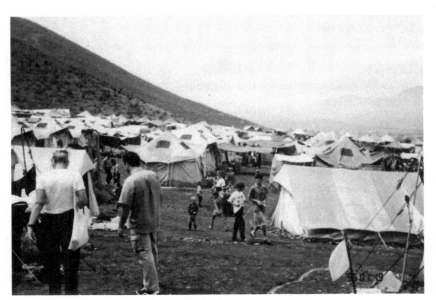

Figure 5.2 Refugees in a camp in Macedonia in 1999.
Reproduced courtesy of John Ashton.

children had been evacuated and transported around the world with over 4000 bound for the United Kingdom, mostly to the North East and North West of England.

Initially, the refugees were in large mixed family groups, sometimes of 10–15 people, some with serious health problems. The main issues were psychological to do with the very stressful experiences and physical and emotional exhaustion. The evacuees were met with overwhelming hospitality in the main and the interagency arrangements of social work, health, housing, and social security worked well. At the very point when I arrived to relieve Nick in Skopje on 9th June the situation changed dramatically with the signing of a peace agreement between the NATO and Yugoslavian forces, and with it an immediate change of direction of the humanitarian effort.

The peace agreement was signed on Friday 10th June with still in excess of 100,000 refugees in the camps inside Macedonia. Once the peace had been agreed, almost immediately the national humanitarian delegations began to withdraw and their operations to run down despite there still being many camp dwellers with health problems, some of them serious. Reports were coming in of the dreadfully degraded state of the health care system in Kosovo itself and, despite the best efforts of the international non-governmental organizations providing care in the camps, they were unable to provide the specialist interventions that many still needed urgently.

Despite the best efforts of the WHO in setting up a disease surveillance system for monitoring the health of the refugees, there was no decent overarching situation analysis. At the daily meetings of the United Nations High Commission on Refugees attention switched to obtaining a picture of the urgent cases in the camps and finding ways to maintain the engagement of country delegations to evacuate those in medical need for a while longer. Together, we spent the weekend agreeing a clear set of criteria for classifying patients for priority medical evacuation, and then embarked on a hectic process of reviewing case notes and other recorded information, sifting and reviewing them as we went to each of the eight camps. By the Sunday night we were left with a single-page summary together with additional analysis by camp, location, and severity as the basis for further mobilization and evacuation (see Box 5.10).

Armed with this information it was possible for us each to make representations to our home governments and through the international bodies to develop a coherent approach to this new phase of the humanitarian emergency. There were four components to this plan:

+ Maintaining adequate primary health care within the camps until all the refugees could return home;

Box 5.10 Review of priority medical cases

Total number of priority cases, 781

  Urgent priority, 311
  Second priority, 326

The most frequent need for treatment

- Reconstructive surgery/orthopaedic/war Injuries, 64
- Oncology/diagnostics/surgery/chemotherapy/radiotherapy, 73
- Haemodialysis, 38
- Congenital malformations requiring orthopaedic intervention, 22
- Endocrinology cases mostly thyrotoxicosis, 17
- Children requiring heart surgery, 9 (other cardiac surgery, 27)
- Psychiatry/neurology including untreated epilepsy; not including war psycho-trauma, 102

- Maintaining medical supplies (in particular insulin, anti-epileptic drugs, and painkillers) with robust logistic supply chains to clinicians;
- Providing additional specialist staff and services to provide support to local hospitals with continuing medical evacuation as needed; and
- Ensuring effective collaboration between agencies and national delegations in the process of rebuilding capacity in the Kosovan health and healthcare systems.

Nick Gent was to play an important part in this last point, returning to Kosovo for a lengthy period in the aftermath of the war and playing a key role in re-establishing the public health system, in particular setting up an effective cold chain to catch up on neglected childhood immunization. By chance a few days later I found myself face to face with President Clinton who was visiting one of the refugee camps and was able to use my two and a half minutes with the President to persuade him to evacuate half the remaining urgent medical cases to the United States (see Box 5.11).

The year 2000, a civil protest brings the country to a halt with impacts on public health

In the lead-up to New Year's Eve, at the dawn of the new millennium, there were widespread fears that computer systems might crash around the world.

Box 5.11 Two and a half minutes with the President

'Coming face to face with President Clinton, the "Have you got a minute, I need to talk to you about the remaining priority medical cases in the camps?" Being met by the totally unexpected "Go on then, tell me about it", and you have 2.5 minutes to tell the tale. At that moment (in touch with emotion and intuition) and in real time it felt like Owen Meaney in John Irving's novel; as if one's entire career to date had been in preparation for this moment—get it right and you can leverage out significant humanitarian assistance at a critical moment, get it wrong and hundreds of people's health and lives may be severely affected. In the novel, Owen Meaney had practised and practised the basketball manoeuvre that, because of his small physique, enabled him to be lifted to score the goal; when the basketball became a grenade in a crowded public space, he was able to throw it through a high-set window. It depended on teamwork and practice, practice coupled with instinct at the critical moment when my local translator, wedged in the crowd, sensed me behind him, eyes in the back of his head, and created a space for me to shake the President's hand and meet his eyes. On that day in Macedonia, and subsequently, I have thought many times of Owen Meaney (and also of Slobodan's example of hands on public health).' (10)

Significant resources were dedicated to ensuring that the worst could not happen and when nothing did, there were recriminations about money wasted. It was reminiscent of those two men on a train in Africa and the non-appearance of the elephants as well as the response to the World Health Organization's declaration of a global flu emergency in 2009. Being between a rock and a hard place when it comes to prevention, you can be damned if you do and damned if you don't in efforts to make it visible. In the North West at least there was a beneficial spin-off from all the work done to prevent a millennial meltdown.

Each winter, from December through until the beginning of spring, the National Health Service was on alert with a team gathered together in an incident room to produce daily 'sitreps' (situation reports). This was to prepare for the winter pressures of cold conditions and increased hospital admissions, with patients waiting on trolleys and in corridors to be seen by a clinician or to find a bed. Meanwhile, the public health team would periodically initiate an incident or outbreak meeting with a separately convened team to monitor the impact of a public health threat. In December 1999, the decision was taken in the North West to integrate these two functions as part of the millennium response. This decision proved to be fortuitous when the nation was brought to a halt by fuel protests in September 2000.

The immediate cause of the fuel protests in the United Kingdom was the rising cost of petrol and diesel fuel for road vehicle use. This was having a particularly severe impact on the farming and rural community. In a move that took government by surprise and inspired by successful earlier protests in France, about 100 farmers and lorry drivers from Wales and the North West of England blockaded the Shell oil refinery at Stanlow in Cheshire. Beginning on Thursday 7th September the protest swept the country with a particular focus on the handful of refineries that produced most of the nation's fuel and by the following Tuesday the country was grinding to a halt with over 3000 filling stations being without fuel. The protests were led by two farmers who hoped to keep the public on side by providing fuel to 'essential users' including hospital medical consultants. However, our sitreps were now telling a fuller and more worrying story and as director of public health, fully briefed about the impact of the dispute on the health and wellbeing of the people of the North West, I was deployed to Stanlow to confront the protestors.

Having made an initial visit to the Stanlow site on the Tuesday evening for an interview with Sky Television News, the interviewers suggested that I return the following morning when the demonstrators would be present in force. With dawn breaking the following morning I found myself confronted by a heckling crowd as, armed with a single sheet of paper, I informed the nation and the world of the impact that the actions of a well-intentioned group was having;

◆ Hospital pharmacies running out of essential medicines because of a 'just in time' approach to holding only 24-hour stocks;

◆ Operating theatre sessions being cancelled in hospitals;

◆ Community nurses in rural areas being unable to attend terminally ill patients in their homes; and

◆ Funeral directors having insufficient petrol to bury the dead.

More generally I was able to point out that the whole idea that it was possible to identify and single out surgeons and hospital consultants as essential workers who could be allowed limited amounts of fuel was misguided, but that hospital cleaners, porters, and operating theatre technicians as well as clerks and cooks were as essential to looking after patients as were the clinicians.

To my absolute amazement, one of the protest leaders immediately announced that he was giving up the protest and going home. In the next hour I was able to speak with several dozen oil tanker drivers in the refinery canteen who had been frightened to take their vehicles out on the road because of violence by some of the crowd outside. Again, they were persuaded by the data I shared with them that they had a social responsibility greater than their concerns for personal safety and within hours the oil supplies were moving out and around the country. During the rest of the day the action crumbled and the country began to return to normal. As I was going into the local radio station in Liverpool late that evening to do one final interview my phone rang; it was Health Minister Alan Milburn to tell me that Prime Minister Blair had asked him to thank me for my intervention. Remembering Slobodan's example I reflected on the privilege it can be to use the platform that public health can offer for the public good when backed up by solid data.

Be wary of water, drownings, and floods, a rising tide but also a slow burn

In many parts of the world water is an ever-present threat to public health, especially through storms and flooding and increasingly as a result of global warming. An unusual example of the hazards of water occurred on the evening of 5 February 2004 at Morecambe Bay in the North West of England when at least 21 Chinese undocumented labourers were drowned whilst picking cockles off the Lancashire coast; they had been illegally employed by a local man and his son. The desperation of their families far away in Fujian province in China can only be imagined but in this incident it was possible to enlist the help of Liverpool public health paediatrician and leader of the local Chinese community, Lord Michael Chan, in establishing links with the victims' home province. Such mental health interventions are often an under-appreciated aspect of disasters.

More conventional disasters involving water began to impact on the North West in the new years of the millennium, the counties of Cumbria and Lancashire being especially vulnerable in view of their topography and location between the waters of the Atlantic Ocean and Irish Sea and the Pennine Mountain range. Beginning in 2004 a succession of floods occurred in different parts of Cumbria, in particular (Kendal, February 2004; Kendal and Carlisle, January 2005; Cockermouth, Keswick, Workington, 2009; with widespread flooding across the whole county with Storm Desmond in December 2015). These floods were subsequently attributed to a number of factors including global warming but also the overgrazing of mountain sides by sheep, leading to excessively fast run-off of rain in heavy storms, the confluence of heavy rain with a high tide on the river Solway in the case of Carlisle, and a failure of drainage maintenance on the lower levels. There were fatalities on a number of occasions, three in 2005, one in 2009, and two in 2015. However, the mental health impact of such events is profound and can be long lasting. The combination of the rupture of personal space and disruption of everyday life together with the unpleasant impact and threat to health of sewage-contaminated living quarters may be compounded by the slow response of insurance companies and the difficulty in securing remedial building work in a reasonable time. Following these incidents it was not uncommon for people to be unable to return to live in their homes for over a year. On the positive side severe environmental events such as flooding tend to impact on all social groups equally and can elicit a strong sense of social solidarity and community cohesion.

Solidarity in floods—the case of Cockermouth

Cockermouth in the north of Cumbria is a charming ancient market town of 10,000 people, popular with second-home owners and retirees. It is situated in the Lake District's northern fells at the confluence of the rivers Cocker and Derwent. Between Wednesday 18th November and Friday 20th, 2009, up to 372 mm of rain fell over the county, being particularly heavy over the up-lying areas and running off rapidly as a result of the ground being already saturated from previous rain. Within a short time the town centre was inundated to a level of several feet with commercial premises and public buildings being flooded out. A major incident was declared and the multiagency response kicked in with the emergency services activated to ensure public safety; fortunately, there was no loss of life. What was particularly impressive was the level of community self-organization, much of which centred on the local health centre and cottage hospital which was in a safer position on higher ground. The local family doctor, John Howarth, with many years of experience in overseas development and disaster areas was instrumental in convening a primary care-led 'Gold' Health Command which brought together members of an extended primary care team, of around 60 people, on a regular basis to assess the situation, apportion responsibilities, and take action to ensure complete continuity of health and social care.

There was initially a complete wipeout of the services for 15,000 people with a loss of two town centre family medicine practices together with both pharmacies along with their stocks of medicines. The prompt action of the clinical staff in retrieving computers through chest high water to the cottage hospital meant that the patient records were safeguarded and clinical care was re-provisioned for the whole town from the one intact facility. A spin-off of the emergency was the bringing together of several clinical teams for the whole town population that had until then been working separately.

With the acute phase over, the community organization which it had generated was well placed to support the recovery phase and to act to minimize adverse long-term effects through contamination and infection and by providing support to fellow citizens in their distress and disruption. In all this was an impressive example of primary care-led leadership and an asset-based approach to a serious community emergency.

Transport deaths, a threat to everyday life

We are so accustomed to the daily toll of deaths and injuries from road traffic collisions that it is quite easy to overlook their significance as public health threats especially in younger people. For example in Cumbria, a county of 500,000 people, in 2006 there were 68 deaths between the ages of 19 and 34, of whom 14 were in motor vehicle crashes. Generally speaking, incidents involving mass passenger transit are much less frequent but when they do occur they have the potential to involve many more people and when these are young people the ramifications can be considerable. In my time in Cumbria over a period of 6 years we experienced two such incidents, one involving a train on the West Coast Main Line between London and Glasgow, the other a school bus on the regular school run at Keswick.

The Grayrigg train derailment and the Keswick school bus crash

The Grayrigg derailment was a fatal incident occurring on a winter's night in open countryside north of the Lake District town of Kendal. It occurred as a result of a faulty set of points that had not undergone their routine inspection. This incident occurred in the early days following yet another National Health Service reorganization with its inevitable loss of corporate memory and self-imposed weaknesses in resilience. The derailment happened at 20.15 on 23 February 2007 and I became aware of it from a Sky television news flash. I immediately contacted the county's hospitals to check that they were prepared for casualties only to discover that this was the first they had heard of the incident. Fortunately, we were able to retrieve the situation and the county's emergency services kicked in efficiently along with a remarkable community response in which 500 first responders turned out to the crash site and provided hot tea and succour to the passengers at a local village school. There was tragically one fatality of an elderly woman and a number of serious injuries. This experience galvanized the NHS in the county into making sure that it was ready for the next time.

The next time was to be three years later when a car collided with a school bus carrying 35 children home from their Keswick school. The bus overturned, killing the car driver and two children, with four more seriously injured. The major incident multiagency response was uneventful, involving multiple ambulances and air ambulances together with the mountain rescue teams, fire engines, and police as casualties were transferred to specialist hospital facilities in towns and cities across the North of England.

Incidents like this are fortunately rare but they must always be used as learning opportunities, especially through post-incident debriefs and audits that look not only at within service but between service functioning. In a sense the coroner holds the key to the final audit, but it has always seemed to me that we don't make enough of the opportunity of collaborating with the local media to spell out the storyline of avoidable factors and the wide-ranging impacts of premature death and life-changing injury. This is especially true in the regular carnage involving young drivers.

Other environmental threats to public health

The natural environment in itself contains many hazards for human populations and the story of mankind has been one of a search for safe habitats with access to food and water. The advent of urbanization created new problems as a result of high population densities and overcrowding with the occurrence of slum conditions predisposing to infectious disease outbreaks. Industrialization added other forms of pollution, including chemicals, other toxic substances, and later radiation. The capacity of humans to soil their own nests is equalled only by their ability to respond to the threats so-caused when motivated and organized. In 1962 Rachel Carson published her dramatic indictment of the chemical industry, *Silent Spring*, in which she accused the industry of spreading misinformation and public officials of accepting industry claims without question. At about the same time Alsatian philosopher Albert Schweitzer summarized the threat succinctly: 'Man has lost the capacity to foresee and to forestall, he will end by destroying the world' (11). Carson's book led to a ban on the agricultural use of DDT and to the establishment of the United States Environmental Agency, and arguably kick started the modern environmentalist movement with its emphasis on ecological as opposed to the more mechanistic sanitary thinking in which out of sight can mean out of mind. In contrast, ecological thinking emphasizes the importance of looking after the things that look after us and not handing on a less sustainable future to the next generation. More recently, commentators have labelled the current geological era as the 'Anthropocene' in which for the first time humans are having a fundamental impact on the viability of the planet Earth. Against this background there are recurrent issues which become part of the work of public health practitioners, issues which may have origins stretching back many years with difficult causal chains to unravel, whilst others may be more recent but nevertheless taxing in the absence of good data but with multifactorial situations and a political environment.

The impact of long-term environmental factors on health

Not infrequently public health departments will be approached by local residents who are concerned about what they perceive to be clusters of health-related events such as congenital abnormalities or cancers. The assumption may be that this should be a relatively easy matter to resolve when in fact it is likely to throw up a paucity of data, questions of historic exposure over many years, and the technical difficulty of making statistical sense of small numbers. Sometimes, as in the case of occupational hazards such as wood dust in the furniture industry and its link to nasal carcinoma or asbestos and its link to mesothelioma, there is robust information on cohorts of workers that can be mined to generate secure cause-and-effect conclusions. Both these examples relate to work carried out by Sir Donald Acheson before he became Chief Medical Officer for England.

A more typical example is illustrated by the findings of a study of industrial atmospheric pollution, historical land use patterns, and mortality which a group of us carried out in the old industrial areas around Liverpool in the early 1990s. By using Standardized Mortality Ratios the 22 local government wards containing the largest proportion of industrial land were compared with the 60 wards with no industrial land, having matched for deprivation. A greater proportion of industrial land in a ward was associated with a higher mortality of ward residents after controlling for the level of socioeconomic deprivation of the residents but that was about as far as it was possible to go with the evidence that was readily available. Situations such as this can be frustrating to local residents and to public health researchers alike and the communication of findings requires a good working relationship with the media to ensure accurate interpretation, especially when it comes to the difficult concept that 'no evidence of an effect is not evidence of no effect'.

A particularly contentious example of an environmental threat to health which has complex political aspects is that of nuclear radiation and nuclear power. There has been concern about the possible adverse health impact of nuclear processes from the earliest days of domestic energy production, starting with a major incident involving the leakage of radioactive liquor from the Windscale plant in Cumbria on 15 March 1979 and subsequent incidents involving accidental releases from the renamed Sellafield plant. Concerns have particularly focused on the possibilities of increased incidence of childhood cancers, hereditary disorders, and stillbirths. In 1990, Martin Gardener, a colleague of Sir Donald Acheson at the Environmental Epidemiology Research Unit at Southampton, reported that the raised incidence of childhood cancers (leukaemia and non-Hodgkin's lymphoma) among children living near to Sellafield was associated with employment of their fathers at Sellafield, and that the association was particularly strong for those whose fathers had received a high dose prior to conception; findings that continue to be contested. The Sellafield context includes a highly political set of factors relating to the continuing national defence dependency on Trident nuclear submarines which are built in Barrow-in-Furness nearby to Sellafield, both industries offering highly paid work in an area of longstanding industrial decline, high unemployment, and otherwise low wages. In addition a lack of credibility of the nuclear industry has been reinforced by its history of retaining the body parts of former nuclear workers for scientific tests without the consent of relatives (see Box 5.12).

Violence as a public health issue

Violence between people is a leading cause of death and disability around the world. Since the end of the Second World War in Europe the continent had been almost free from military and paramilitary violence until the civil war in former Yugoslavia. Since then such forms of conflict have once again become major threats to public health. The 11 September 2001 attacks by the terrorist group al-Qaeda on the United States marked a new phenomenon in mass terrorism and civilian casualties with 2,977 deaths, predominantly of civilians and New York firemen. Subsequent international developments with the second Gulf War in 2003, the spread of Islamic fundamentalist terrorism, and the displacement of large civilian populations from countries including Syria have changed the world's politics and how we live and served to ensure that emergency planning is prominent on government and public health radar. Following these events and in response to the climate of fear and increasing levels of hate crime in local communities, we used the standing of the office of Regional Director of Public Health to establish a dialogue between the different faith communities of the region under the rubric of 'Common Ground'.

However, important as it is, armed conflict between military, paramilitary, and terrorist groups is not the only type. In 2002, the World Health Organization published its seminal report on *World Violence and Health*. This comprehensive review defined and measured the extent of the problem in member states and drew attention to the fact that when it came to prevention, violence was essentially an orphan. Whilst Home Offices and police departments might be

Box 5.12 The Chernobyl nuclear disaster, 26 April 1986

The Chernobyl nuclear accident is one of only two reported level 7 nuclear accidents (nine being the maximum), the other being that in Fukushima in Japan in 2011. Design flaws during a reactor test led to an uncontrolled reaction, a destructive steam explosion, and fire followed by nine days in which nuclear fission products were released across the west of the Soviet Union and Europe. The reactor has been enclosed in a large sarcophagus radiation shield ever since, the surrounding population having been permanently evacuated.

During the immediate incident there were 2 deaths within the plant and later 29 firemen died from acute radiation syndrome with unknown numbers subsequently affected. On a professional visit to Cuba in 2013 I was told that thousands of children from the Chernobyl area had been treated in Cuba for thyroid cancer.

Shortly after the disaster I was working with public health colleagues in Sweden who told me that all Swedes had been required to destroy any vegetables that they were growing in their gardens. This was not the case in the UK although hill farmers in parts of the north west of England and Wales were prohibited from selling their sheep for consumption, a prohibition that apparently continues 30 years later. Whilst visiting Spain the same year, a colleague recommended Welsh lamb in the restaurant as it was 'currently very cheap'!

The difficulty of demonstrating causality in questions like these and in the more general matter of the impact of the long-term exposure to low levels of harmful risks in the environment cannot be overstated. It is important to start from the ancient premise of 'Primum non Nocere', or at the least to do no harm and to remember that no firm evidence of no effect is not the same as evidence of no effect.

responsible for apprehending and punishing the perpetrators of crimes against the person and whilst health services might pick up the pieces in terms of treatment, who was responsible for reducing the toll in the first place?

Seven categories of violence were identified in the WHO report and along with it came a recommendation and a programme of international policy development to encourage the acceptance of shared responsibility for prevention between crime and health agencies (see Box 5.13).

Box 5.13 Categories of violence (WHO, 2002)

- Youth violence
- Child abuse and neglect by parents and other caregivers
- Violence by intimate partners
- Abuse of the elderly
- Sexual violence
- Self-directed violence
- Collective violence

Following the publication of the WHO report and its discussion with UK Chief Medical Officer Liam Donaldson, the North West Public Health Observatory under Mark Bellis took on a lead role on behalf of the CMO. As a result, the Centre for Public Health at Liverpool John Moores University became a collaborating centre with the World Health Organization Geneva office for research and development into public health approaches to violence prevention. The collaborating centre drew on the experience of the Centres for Disease Control in Atlanta to publish a British version of the WHO report 'Violent Britain—People, Prevention and Public Health' and held a national conference to raise the issues of violence as a public health issue. This was formative not just for the UK but on a wider basis with the production, with WHO, of international guidance on the primary prevention of violence. By the time of yet another NHS reorganization in 2013, when the base for local public health in England was returned to local authorities, local directors of public health had an identified lead role for violence prevention in their communities.

Mass shootings in the countryside: a mental health emergency

At 10.13 am on 2 June 2010, a local taxi driver on the west coast of Cumbria, Derrick Bird, went on a rampage with a 12-gauge double-barrelled shotgun and a 22 calibre bolt-action rifle. By the time he had finished a spree in a rural area that created 30 different crime scenes and he was found dead in a wooded area, 12 people were dead and 11 seriously injured. The event was the most serious in the United Kingdom since the Dunblane school massacre in Scotland in 1996 in which 18 people were killed. The victims were largely shot at random and at close range and there was never subsequently a clear explanation as to what the motivation had been.

At the time these events were unfolding I was attending the annual WHO violence prevention business meeting in Rome and took a phone call from my lead on health protection, Nigel Calvert. After discussion with Rodney Hammond, Director of the Division of Violence Prevention at the Centers for Disease Control in Atlanta, Georgia, it was immediately apparent that rather than returning to the major incident centre in Cumbria it would make more sense to draw on Rodney's experience and feed in his recommendations over the phone. Rodney's view was that the immediate incident would be over in a few hours, which was indeed the case, the gunman having killed himself and the seriously injured having been flown by helicopter to trauma centres across the North of England. The advice I was given was that this was best treated as a mental health emergency and that attention should now focus on the first responders and bystanders.

My philosophy as a public health director was always to drink regular coffee with the chief police and fire officers and other key leaders so that in emergencies the relationships were on a sound footing. I enjoyed a particularly good relationship with Cumbria Chief Constable Craig Mackie and was able to share Rodney's wisdom over the phone. Within hours we had put in place 24/7 access to counselling for those who would need it, knowing at the same time, from experience elsewhere, that comparatively few would avail themselves of it. By the time I returned home a day or so later Craig was ready to hand over the Gold Command chair to myself as public health director to deal with the longer term mental health fallout.

We ran that Gold Command for over a year. During this time we put in place low-key enhanced surveillance in cooperation with faith and local political leaders, family doctors, schoolteachers, social workers, the voluntary sector, and many others, including the police. A data base of 2000 first responders and bystanders to the awful events of 2nd June was the basis for keeping a watchful eye on our communities and also reaching out to the home bases of those tourists who had been passing through the county at the time and been caught up in the emergency. We were able to identify a significant number of people, including several dozen children who were suffering from post-traumatic stress and enable them to receive the therapeutic support that they needed.

Understanding apparently random outbreaks of extreme violence such as that perpetrated by Derrick Bird can be difficult. In the context of the violence that has occurred over many years in central and South America, our colleague

Alberto Concha Eastman has described an interconnected three-tiered model. At the top are the structural factors such as socioeconomic inequality, poverty, corruption, political instability, human rights violations, and rapid urbanization. The second tier relates to institutional factors such as a lack of public confidence in the police and judicial system, leading to a poor sense of security and protection, low levels of education, poor parenting, and family breakdown. The final level includes the facilitating or direct factors which may trigger or lead to catastrophic events. Alcohol and narcotic consumption have been strongly associated with homicide, violent injuries, and domestic violence and the ready availability of guns facilitates their use.

Since the steady spate of mass killings in schools began in the United States with the Columbine massacre on 20 April 1999, attention has also been focused on contagious aspects and the role of mass and social media, which can also be an issue with outbreaks of suicide. Four weeks after the Cumbria shootings, not far away in Northumberland, another man, 37-year-old Raoul Moat, who had recently been released from Durham Prison, shot three people in two days before going on the run. Cornered by the police, he shot himself. Many commentators at the time believed that the extensive and sensationalistic press reporting of the previous Derrick Bird murders must have played a part.

As public health director with a longstanding interest in the contagious aspects of murder and suicide, I took the opportunity of once again lobbying the Press Complaints Commission about their code of practice on reporting such occurrences with limited effect and in the aftermath I was called to give evidence to the House of Commons Home Office Select Committee. My evidence to the committee addressed the issue of firearms control and the role of family doctors in vetting applicants for gun licences. My suggestion was that rather than keeping the status quo in which personal physicians could be in the uncomfortable position of having to object to a licence for one of their own patients, it would make more sense to have a panel of doctors who were able to develop a special interest in the matter. Unfortunately, there continues to be a complacency about such matters, although the problem is much less than in some other countries.

Protecting the public health in the digital age

Almost 30 years after the end of the Cold War between the Soviet Union and the Western Block we have entered a new era of global economics and trade, mass global mobility and travel, and diffuse and new forms of global insecurity. One of the primary functions of government remains the protection of its citizens either from external threats from hostile forces and internal threats from anti-social and criminal behaviour or from the forces of nature. New forms of global social media have added a novel layer of complexity and have brought with them the potential for enhancing health and wellbeing but also the capacity to undermine it and to the detriment of national and economic security and mental health. The new tensions between freedom and security are evident in contemporary debates that include, for example, the policing of online access to pornography and the safety of our children. We have barely scratched the surface of an adequate response to the safeguarding of children and other vulnerable groups in this new situation.

One issue that this new era has thrown up is the limits to professional solutions which depend on the specialist expertise of particular groups of workers. In my time as a director of public health in Cumbria we were confronted by a series of catastrophic failures to safeguard the county's children which resulted in deaths and serious injury. A system that was heavily dependent on the professional expertise of social workers and others to protect the vulnerable was repeatedly found wanting. Efforts to encourage cross-agency working could not break through the siloed boundaries of professional jealousies. In particular there was a failure to recognize that the notion that 'it takes a village to raise a child 'is at least as relevant today in the age of global social media as it was when children went to the village school, transport was by horse and cart, and mail was infrequent. There will never be enough social workers, child psychiatrists, or other experts to protect and defend the vulnerable. With perhaps two billion people accessing electronic media worldwide there will never be enough policemen to police the Net; it must be down to the users themselves acting in concert in the same way that the future of health and health care must be by co-production. We need widespread expertise as much as experts and active citizens who recognize a responsibility to look out for children and others who are vulnerable outside their own families. In the Internet age the power for good through mass education must be at least as great as the power for harm. Community resilience and the prevention of harm is too important to be left to professional elites.

When I began my public health career the dominant approach to health emergency planning in the shadow of the Cold War was by and large to keep the public in the dark. I have contested this for over 30 years and hope to have played a part in bringing it out of the closet using public health annual reports (see Figure 5.3). I am pleased to report that by the time I stepped down from my role in Cumbria in 2013 the county emergency plan, with minimal redactions, was available on the Internet.

Personal Resilience Guide

County Council   Cumbria

Prepare for an Emergency

To prepare for an emergency, you should take time to find out:

- Where and how to turn off water, gas and electricity supplies in your home
- The emergency procedures for your children at school and at your workplace
- How your family will stay in contact in the event of an emergency
- If any elderly or vulnerable neighbours might need your help
- How to tune in to your local radio station
- Fit and maintain smoke alarms in your home and plan an escpare route should a fire break out
- Be aware of important supplies you may need in an emergency such as prescribed medication, candles and spare clothes.

What to do in an Emergency

If you find yourself in the middle of an emergency, your common sense and instincts will usually tell you what to do. However, it is important to:

- Make sure **999** has been called if people are injured or if there is a threat to life
- Not put yourself or others in danger
- Follow the advice of the emergency services
- Try to remain calm and think before acting, and try to reassure others
- Check for injuries - remember to help yourself before attempting to help others.

If you are not involved in the incident, but are close by or believe you may be in danger, in most cases the advice is:

- Go inside a safe building
- Stay inside until you are advised to do otherwise
- Tune in to local radio or TV for more information.

Of course, there are always going to be particular occasions when you should not "go in" to a building, for example if there is a fire. Otherwise:

GO IN, STAY IN, TUNE IN.

Basic First Aid

Knowing some basic first aid skills could help you deal with an emergency – your relatives or friends could be the ones to benefit from your skills.

When there is more than one injured person, go to the quietest one first.

They may be unconscious and need immediate attention.

Learning first aid is easy so why not take a few minutes now to familiarise yourself with the first aid scenarios below, or enrol on a basic first aid course.

Unconscious

If the casualty is not responding but is able to breathe normally, turn them onto their side to protect their airway. If there are no signs of life, call 999 and ask for an ambulance. Follow the call handlers advice on how to give chest compressions and mouth-to-mouth resuscitations while you wait for the ambulance to arrive.

Severe bleeding

Control severe bleeding by applying firm pressure to the wound using a clean, dry dressing and raise it above the level of the heart. Lay the person down, reassure them, keep them warm and loosen tight clothing.

Burns

For all burns, cool with water for at least 10 minutes. Wrap the affected part in clingfilm, do not apply dry dressings, keep the patient warm and call an ambulance.

Broken Bones

Try to cause as little movement as possible.

Choking

Encourage the casualty to cough if they are able to do so. If not, lean them forward and give up to five sharp blows between the shoulder blades. If this fails, give up to five thrusts in the stomach if you or a bystander have the skills to do this.

Emergency Contact Details

Compile a list of useful emergency contact numbers and keep them somewhere easily accessible to you – on your fridge door for example.

Emergency services:	999
NHS Direct:	0845 46 47
Anti terrorist hotline:	0800 789 321
Cumbria Constabulary:	**Non Emergency Number - 101** (available 24 hours a day, 7 days a week).
Cumbria County Council:	01228 606060

Local District Council:	
Doctor:	
Work:	
Schools:	
Family contact 1:	
Family contact 2:	
Local Radio Station & Frequency:	

Figure 5.3 Personal Resilience Guide for Cumbria 2011. The Annual Report of the Director of Public Health.

Reproduced from Cumbria 2011: The Annual Report of the Director of Health. NHS Cumbria. © Crown Copyright.

References

1. **Neumann, S.** *Die Offentliches Gesundheitstflege und das eigenthum.* Berlin, 1847. Quoted in **H. Sigerist,** *Medicine and Human Welfare.* Oxford: Oxford University Press, 1941.

2. **World Health Organization.** *International Statistical Classification of Diseases and Related Health Problems,* 10th revised version, Chapter 20. Geneva: WHO, 2006.

3. **Ashton, John.** Pollution of the water supply in Mersey and Clwyd—a cause for concern? *Community Medicine* **7** (1985), 299–303.

4. **The Final Report of the UK Drug Policy Commission.** *A Fresh Approach to Drugs* (2012).

5. **Fowler, Norman.** *AIDS, Don't Die of Prejudice.* London: Biteback Publishing, 2014.

6. **Shilts, Randy.** *And The Band Played On: Politics, People and the AIDS Epidemic.* New York: St Martin's Press, 1987.

7. **Acheson, Sir Donald.** *Public Health in England: The Report of the Committee of Inquiry into the Future Development to the Public Health Function.* London: HM Stationary Office, 1988.

8. **BBC.com.** 1988: Egg industry fury over salmonella claim. *On This Day, 1950–2005.* Available at: http://news.bbc.co.uk/onthisday/hi/dates/stories/december/3/newsid_2519000/2519451.stm.

9. **Ashton, J.** Balkans briefing number 5. Seeking refuge (Macedonia, 9–25 June 1999): The changing needs of humanitarian aid in the face of the peace. *Journal of Epidemiology and Community Health* **54**(6) (2000), 469–72.

10. **Ashton, John. R.** Two and a half minutes with the President. *Journal of Epidemiology and Community Health* **54**(9) (2000), 708.

11. **Carson, Rachel.** *Silent Spring.* New York: Houghton Mifflin, 1962.

Further Reading

Advice about Vaccination Policy in Boarding Schools. *A Joint BSA and MOSA Guideline for Head Teachers.* Boarding Schools Association, Faculty of Public Health, Medical Officers of Schools Association, 2014.

Agendas for Change. *Environmental Health Commission.* London: Chartered Institute for Environmental Health, 1997.

Ashton, John. Pollution of the water supply in Mersey and Clwyd—a cause for concern? *Community Medicine* **7** (1985), 299–303.

Ashton, John. Sanitarian becomes ecologist: the new environmental health. sensitivity to the environment demands new skills and attitudes. *British Medical Journal* **302** (1991), 189–90.

Ashton, J. Balkans briefing number 5. Seeking refuge (Macedonia, 9–25 June 1999): The changing needs of humanitarian aid in the face of the peace. *Journal of Epidemiology and Community Health* **54**(6) (2000), 469–72.

Ashton, John. R. Two and a half minutes with the President. *Journal of Epidemiology and Community Health* **54**(9) (2000), 708.

Ashton, John R. Book of the month: *War or Health?* Book review. *Journal of the Royal society of Medicine* **95** (2002), 214–15.

Ashton, John. 'If Ebola was in the UK we'd cure it,' says leading doctor. *Independent on Sunday*, 3 August 2014.

Ashton, John R., and Seymour Howard. Public Health and the origins of the Mersey Model of harm reduction. *International journal of Drug Policy* **21**(2) (2010): 94–6.

Barry, John M. *The Great Influenza: The Epic Story of the Deadliest Plague in History.* London: Viking Penguin, 2004.

Bennett, E., M. Ashton, N. Calvert, J. Chaloner, J. Cheesbrough, J. Egan, et al. Barrow-in Furness: a large community legionellosis outbreak in the UK. *Epidemiology and Infection* **142** (2014)., 1763–77.

Byerly. Carol R. *Fever of War: The Influenza Epidemic in the U.S. Army during World War 1.* New York: New York University Press, 2005.

Carson, Rachel. *Silent Spring.* New York: Houghton Mifflin, 1962.

Concha-Eastman, A. Violence: a challenge for public health and for all. *Journal of Epidemiology and Community Health* **55** (2001), 597–9.

Convert, I., and C. Bailey. After the flood: the health and social consequences of the 2005 Carlisle flood event. *Journal of Flood Risk Management* **1** (2008), 100–9.

de Alarcon, R. The spread of heroin abuse in a community. United Nations Office on drugs and Crime. *Bulletin on Narcotics*, **Issue 3** (1969), 1–9.

Fowler, Norman. *AIDS, Don't Die of Prejudice.* London: Biteback Publishing, 2014.

France, David. *How to Survive a Plague: The Story of How Activists and Scientists Tamed AIDS.* London: Picador, 2016.

Garrett, Laurie. *Betrayal of Trust: The Collapse of Global Public Health,* New York: Hyperion, 2000.

Health and Safety Executive. *The Leakage of Radioactive Liquor into the Ground, British Nuclear Fuels Limited, Windscale, 15 March 1979.* London: Health and Safety Executive, 1980.Hein, Piet. *Grooks.* Copenhagen: Borgens Forlag, 1974.

Healthy People. *The Surgeon General's Report on Health Promotion and Disease Prevention.* Background Papers. Washington, DC: US Department of Health, Education, and Welfare, 1979.

Irving, John. *A Prayer for Owen Meany.* New York: William Morrow, 1989.

Jones, Lisa, Geoff Bates, Ellie McCoy, Olivia Wording, Jim McVeigh, and Mark Bellis. *Positive and Negative Impacts of the Nuclear Industry on Health and Well-Being.* Liverpool: Centre for Public Health, Liverpool John Moores University, 2011.

Kevin Sampson in association with the Hillsborough Justice Campaign. *Hillsborough Voices: The Real Story Told by the People Themselves.* London: Ebury Press, 2016.

McVeigh, Clare, K. Hughes, Mark A. Bellis, Emma Reed, John R. Ashton, Qutub Syed. *Violent Britain: People, Prevention and Public Health.* Liverpool: Centre for Public Health, Liverpool John Moores University, 2005.

McLaughlin, J., V. Mithani, F. J. Bolton, G. L. Nichols, M. A. Bellis, Q. Syed, et al. An investigation into the microflora of heroin. *Journal of Medical Microbiology* **51** (2002), 1001–8.

Midgely, Jane, Nick Ashton, Helen Castles, Jane McNamara, Karen Tocqueville, and Mark Bellis. *Health, Environment and Deprivation in the North West of England.* Liverpool: Centre for Public Health, Liverpool John Moores University, 2005.

Piot, Peter. *No Time to Lose: A Life in Pursuit of Deadly Viruses.* New York/London: Norton, 2012.

Royal College of Physicians. *Every Breath We Take: The Lifelong Impact of Air Pollution.* London: RCP, 2016.

Sainsbury, Peter, Ruth Hussey, John Ashton, and Boswell Andrews. Industrial atmospheric pollution, historical land use patterns and mortality. *Journal of Public Health Medicine* 18(1) (1996), 87–93.

Shilts, Randy. *And The Band Played On: Politics, People and the AIDS Epidemic.* New York: St Martin's Press, 1987.

The Final Report of the UK Drug Policy Commission. *A Fresh Approach to Drugs* (2012).

Toque, Karen, and M. Bellis (Eds). BSE and Public Health. *Perspectives from Agriculture, Food Policy and Epidemiology.* North West Public Health Association, 1996.

Wilson, D., N. Calvert, and P. Boriello. Editorial: Managing major public health crises: Lessons from recent events in the United States and the United Kingdom. *BMJ* 323 (2000), 1321–2.

World Health Organization. *World Report on Violence and Health.* Geneva: WHO, 2002.

Chapter 6

Population health care

The big picture

In his *British Medical Journal* paper of 1980, Professor Jerry Morris posed the question 'Are health services important to the people's health?' (1). He raised this issue because the idea was spreading that health services were of 'little moment' in the overall scheme of things. He took issue with Thomas McKeown, whose writings on the role of medicine had become influential in the thinking behind the New Public Health. Morris argued that playing down the health service contribution was based on a misconception derived from over-attachment to history and the toll of premature death that accompanied Victorian living conditions. Morris drew attention to the improvements in life expectancy and reducing relevance of the absence of disease as health measures and highlighted the host of 'chronic conditions' currently unpreventable, but where treatment might make all the difference to the quality of life. Advances in scientific medicine since 1980 have reinforced the importance of this message whilst the momentum for prevention has so far failed to rebalance the relative investment in hospital versus community interventions. Having answered this question with a resounding 'yes' only raises another question, namely, 'What is the contribution of public health to health services?'

The public health task is determined by a combination of demography, patterns of ill-health and their determinants, and the availability of policies and interventions which can impact on health outcomes through 'the organized efforts of society'. One such organized effort is the provision of health services themselves and the contribution that public health expertise can offer to their working; the other side of the coin is the contribution of public health to action on health determinants and the mitigation of risk.

Public health specialists bring to the table perspectives and skills that can clarify, frame, and begin to measure and evaluate those interventions, including the evaluation of the contribution of health services. In this sense prevention, treatment, and care are not in opposition but complement each other in a systematic and whole systems way. Epidemiology, an underpinning discipline of public health, has the potential to contribute greatly to this together with the other social, biological, and environmental sciences. Jerry Morris's book *The*

Uses of Epidemiology offers seven potential ways in which the study of epidemiology can shed light on these important matters (see Box 6.1).

The interaction of all seven uses is relevant in understanding how health and healthcare systems work. A narrow approach to community diagnosis concentrating on 'needs', without also taking into account the 'assets' of individuals and communities, risks prescription which is over-dependent on professional solutions and can undermine inherent resilience and coping skills rather than building on them. This becomes a particular problem in understanding the proper role of hospitals and hospital beds in the ecology of health service provision. Typically audits of the bed occupancy of acute hospitals find that perhaps one-third of patients are inappropriately placed compared with what is possible with the right kind of housing stock for supported living, a health literate population, and strong community health and social care. This can include the kind of extended primary care provision to be found especially in parts of Scandinavia. Professor Bob Logan, of the London School of Hygiene and Tropical Medicine, has summed up this dilemma with two of 'Logan's Laws':

1. Logan's First Law: 'You can't grow potatoes in an empty bed', recognizing the inertia that comes from hospital consultants maintaining their sphere of influence within an institutional setting.

2. Logan's Second Law: 'The number of beds you have is the number of beds you need', making explicit a reality that systems develop around fixed structures in defiance of the edict that structure should follow function.

The inertia to change of hospital-based systems of care and their potential for middle-class capture of their function is not new but there are examples of flexing provision to adapt to changing needs. During the cholera outbreaks in Liverpool, Duncan and his colleagues opened temporary clinical facilities

---

Box 6.1 The uses of epidemiology

- Historical study
- Community diagnosis: community health
- Working of health services
- Individual chances and risks
- Identification of syndromes
- Completion of the clinical picture
- In search of causes.

for as long as the need lasted; after the Second World War, with the decline in tuberculosis, many sanatoria were closed and chest physicians retrained; and later the therapeutic optimism engendered by the discovery of psychoactive medicines led to the closure of mental asylums and beds. Most recently the need for specialist beds for AIDS patients came and went with the trajectory of the epidemic and the advent of effective outpatient treatment. Unfortunately, for historic reasons, the provision of health services begins with the provision of institutional care, with hospitals as modern cathedrals hoping to stave off death in a secular age. Efforts at reorientation usually begin with incremental change to the status quo rather than fundamental redesign. Effective redesign must start with population-level health literacy and skills, with pathways via primary care based on the principle of subsidiarity. Care should be provided as close as possible to home as is compatible with the tradeoff between access, quality, and cost. That the starting point should lie with a population possessing health knowledge, skills, and practices resonates with John McKnight's asset-based aphorism that 'you don't go to the store until you have seen what you have in the larder or the backyard'.

Reconciling access, quality, and cost

In the pre-industrial, pre-urban age and before the advent of scientific medicine the emphasis of health and social care was very much grounded in lay and domestic health practices. In his 1975 treatise *Medical Nemesis*, the radical thinker Ivan Illich described 'the expropriation of health' in which an ever-increasing professionalization of the management of everyday conditions was incompatible with affordable, comprehensive health care. The argument is that what is needed is the right balance between expertise and experts.

One might ask how has the remorseless professionalization of lay care come about? For one thing the roll-out of new expertise from experts to generalists and on to the public has largely been absent in medical care in contrast to what is commonplace in other sectors. In the medical field highly trained and expensively paid professionals not only do the research and development but usually continue to provide the individual service themselves. There are examples from the technical end of medicine, for example in the Netherlands, where anaesthetists may oversee anaesthetic technicians in the simultaneous running of more than one operating theatre, or in specific routine surgical operations which may be entrusted to technicians; even here there is often a reluctance by those at the top of the clinical hierarchy to delegate and share expertise. Until recently there has been a monopolization of terminal care of patients by the palliative care 'high priests' with little roll-out of expertise into the community to other clinicians, let alone family members. George Bernard Shaw proposed that 'all professions are conspiracies against the laity'. This is apposite when we consider that the health and social care professions have laid claim to larger and larger tracts of territory which they cannot realistically occupy. This has replaced what has been, and can be again in the age of the Internet, a robust and extensive lay care system underpinned by the expertise of experts with the systematic cascade of new knowledge and skills.

This flaw is understandable within a private practice frame of reference, which has often had undue influence over the structures and governance of public health care systems. Professionals seek to engage with individuals in a transaction for money based on superior knowledge and skills. The more sickness or sickness behaviour there is and demand for services, the better. This does not sit comfortably with a public health frame of reference or with health services dedicated to the equitable provision of care to the whole population. What does make sense is the skilling up of that population and supporting lay health skills. Encouragingly in recent years there are examples, such as in the care of patients with diabetes where the importance of having 'expert patients' has become overwhelming. More generally things are beginning to change as a result of the demographic pressure of an ageing population and pressure on resources, but real co-production in which citizens and clinicians work in democratic tandem has far to go. Philosophically the starting point needs to be that of the psychotherapist trying to do herself out of a job rather than allowing dependency to develop. It may be a matter of enlightened self-interest and is possible. Parts of Finland have reduced general practice consultations by 20 per cent by skilling up the population in dealing with common conditions with no detriment to patient health. In the United Kingdom where there is an end of life gap between patients who wish to die at home and a system which militates against this, there are signs of relatives and 'buddies' being supported with the necessary skills to facilitate good deaths, simultaneously reducing the burden of hospital costs. Initiatives such as 'making every (clinical) contact count' and 'expert patients' are straws in the wind of what should happen.

Perhaps most fundamentally, the integration of town and country planning with health and social care can lead to the right kind of housing investment that facilitates independent living for those with long-term conditions.

What sort of health services do we need?

So what is the vision of a well-functioning, high-quality, affordable health care system that meets the public health imperative of whole population coverage?

For a start we need systems that are grounded in the wider health system, encompassing the settings and functions of everyday life, the places and ways in which health is gained, threatened and lost, or retrieved. In such a system health care is a subset of public health rather than public health being a subset of health care, as so often seems to be assumed. Healthcare is an important part of public health but it contributes only a small part to our health and wellbeing.

The truth of this claim was accepted in the Wanless Report, published in England in 2004 by Sir Derek Wanless in response to the Chancellor of the Exchequer's request to examine the case for more funding for the National Health Service. Funding levels were then lagging behind comparable European country levels and levels of spending on public health and prevention were similarly unequal. At that time NHS investment on prevention and public health spending was about 1.8 per cent compared with 2.5 per cent in France, 4.5 per cent in Germany, and over 5 per cent in the Netherlands.

Sir Derek explored three scenarios as part of his task:

◆ In scenario one the NHS would continue providing care along the same lines with a dominance of hospital-based investment and provision. In this scenario the NHS would be unable to meet its obligation to provide equitable high-quality access to the whole population within 20 years.

◆ In scenario two the NHS would roll out evidence-based best practice from the best performing organizations across the whole health care system but with the same priorities for hospitals, primary and community care, prevention, and public health. Under this scenario the NHS would still fail to meet its obligations but it would take longer.

◆ In the third scenario, described as 'the fully engaged scenario', there would be a fundamental re-orientation away from hospital domination to one in which citizens were fully engaged in matters affecting their own health in a partnership of co-production with clinicians and strong primary and community care. With this approach the viability of the National Health Service and its ability to meet its aims should be safeguarded.

Chancellor of the Exchequer Gordon Brown was persuaded of the arguments put forward by Sir Derek and released significant additional funds. These were subsequently used for a major hospital rebuilding programme and to boost clinical salaries with no long-term impact on the development of public health capacity or resources. Within 10 years the NHS was facing ever-deepening crises exacerbated by the needs of a rapidly ageing population.

So what needs to be done?

Too often a historic legacy of institutional care creates a rigid structure of provision. In the British case the roots of this can be traced right back to the agricultural revolution of the eighteenth century and the displacement of rural peasants from the countryside. Their dispossession and migration to the burgeoning towns and cities created a homelessness problem that was dealt with by the Poor Laws, the creation of workhouses for those without work or shelter, and for the sick poor, the building of workhouse hospitals. Many of these hospitals were absorbed into the National Health Service when it was established in 1948 and over the years have become a fixture of the National Health Service structures. These have often been rebuilt in defiance of the changing needs of a much better housed population made up of smaller, healthier families with changed health needs, and of progressive thinking which has tried with little success to copy the examples of primary care-led health services to be found in some other countries.

A good starting point for an affordable, high-quality, and accessible health care system, grounded within a public health system, would be the eight elements of the Alma Ata Declaration, adopted by the World Health Organization in 1977 (see Box 6.2).

At first glance this list may appear to be of little relevance to so-called developed countries, but it bears closer examination and reflection. It represents a remarkable consensus by ministers of health from countries at different stages of development, is resilient, and is as relevant today as it was 40 years ago.

Box 6.2 The eight elements of the Alma Ata Declaration

- Health education
- Food supply and proper nutrition
- Safe water and basic sanitation
- Maternal and child health care
- Immunization
- Prevention and control of endemic diseases
- Basic treatment of health problems
- Provision of essential drugs

International commitment to the Alma Ata principles was re-confirmed at a global fortieth anniversary conference in Kazakhstan in 2018.

Health education

We have barely scratched the surface of what a meaningful strategy for health education should look like in the Internet age, the coming era of co-production and a redefining of the role of clinical advisers in relation to the public. Before the coming of the National Health Service and before the new technologies those who could not afford to seek medical advice were dependent on where they could find it. My own father with type 1 diabetes in 1937, in a poorly paid job, and with a family to support was not alone in depending on a lay encyclopaedia of health distributed by one of the national newspapers. In the intervening years we have made formal medical care more and more the first port of call for the management of everyday medical problems whilst around us we have neighbourhood pharmacies containing staff with clinical knowledge and skills; a population with widespread access to further and higher education, and an empire of medical knowledge at the press of a button. It is time for us to embrace the magic prospect offered by mass health literacy, health expertise, and self-management. There is scope for a significant shift away from dependency to co-production and self-efficacy.

Food supply and proper nutrition

The food problems of the nineteenth century were usually those of food poverty and food adulteration. Surprisingly things have not really changed much in that food poverty has reappeared in many places with food banks filling the gap for people on low income, whilst a twenty-first-century version of food adulteration characterized by processing with high levels of fat, sugar, and salt have contributed to an international epidemic of obesity, vascular disease, and diabetes. Largely preventable through progressive and enlightened approaches to government policy and intervention in the market, the impact of these trends on ill health and medical care is massive.

Safe water and basic sanitation

Whilst for most people living in more affluent parts of the world, the availability of safe water can be mostly taken for granted, this is not necessarily true for those in poor housing and who struggle to make ends meet in a world of privatized water and other utilities where 'the poor pay the most' in not having access to the cheapest tariffs. Nor, with the recurrence of episodes of water-borne infection such as cryptosporidium, can we be certain that our water is always bacteriologically safe when the interests of shareholders take precedence over those of citizen consumers; and there are longstanding questions over the effect of low levels of chemical pollution in water supplies taken over many years. The impact of global warming on the security of water supplies looks ominous for many especially farmers and growers.

Maternal and child health care

Dramatic global reductions in maternal and child mortality over the past 100 years point to a success story, but it is more complicated than that. The deaths of almost 1000 women every year in childbirth in 1930s England and Wales led to the establishment of the highly effective Confidential Enquiry into Stillbirths and Deaths in Infancy. Within a few decades these numbers were reduced to dozens, most of whom had complicated medical histories. On the other hand, the big rise in morbidly obese and older women is a matter of concern to obstetricians and in an era of very low family size where every pregnancy is special, the pressures to reconcile safe care with patient choice and geographical considerations are one of the most fraught challenges. Social changes including the rise of single parent and non-traditional households and increased mobility have created new challenges for child-raising and with older children there are worries about deteriorating mental health.

Immunization

The blessing of the wide range of immunizations now available for child health and wellbeing would have amazed our grandparents and great grandparents. Yet they have not been universally embraced and children are being put at risk by decisions made on their behalf by adults who carry a duty of care. Handling this situation is one of the real tests of the art and science of the practice of public health.

Prevention and control of endemic diseases

The dynamic nature of the threats to health is well illustrated with reference to their constant shifts, the coming and going, and the need for surveillance, intelligence, and informed responses. In *The Uses of Epidemiology* Morris drew attention to the dramatic decline in tuberculosis, pneumonia, rheumatic heart disease, rickets, and mastoiditis with their replacement by contemporary scourges of ischaemic heart disease and lung cancer. Subsequently, over the past 40 years we have seen the appearance of a whole series of new infectious diseases including HIV/AIDS, BSE, Legionella, and Ebola as well as epidemics of lifestyle and degenerative conditions including diabetes, dementia, and the accumulated conditions which accompany longevity. Keeping abreast of these, getting upstream where possible to prevention, and developing appropriate and sustainable responses for ongoing care is a moving target resembling the layers of an onion, with new challenges being revealed by the disappearance of existing ones.

Basic treatment of health problems

The conundrum, the challenge, and the prize is that of developing coherent approaches to the treatment of basic health problems which optimize self-care, generic and specialist interventions at the right level in the right place and time. Describing, understanding, intervening, and evaluating these problems is a public health task that requires a multi- and interdisciplinary approach.

Provision of essential drugs

Perhaps 10 per cent of National Health Service budgets are spent on pharmaceuticals which may be lifesaving, significantly improve the quality of life, be of dubious benefit or be positively detrimental. Optimizing the use of appropriate medicines requires rational frameworks, evidence-based science, partnerships, and pragmatism. The opportunity costs of getting it wrong are significant.

Public health and primary care

Those countries, such as Finland, that have taken the bold step of redesigning their health system to be grounded in public health and prevention and based on primary care have benefited from it enormously. The Finn Hanna Vuori has argued that there are four ways in which the concept of primary health care can be interpreted:

◆ As a set of activities;

◆ As a level of care;

◆ As a strategy of organizing health care; and

◆ As a philosophy.

The reorientation from primary medical care as a medical concept, albeit involving multidisciplinary teams of health workers based in the community, to primary health care requires a conceptual and practical leap. Primary health care is a social approach based on World Health Organization and public health principles in being concerned with populations as well as individuals and seeking to involve a range of people in addition to trained health workers; it seeks partnership with the public and with community associations. In making the step from primary medical care it reaches out to make the connections between the determinants of health and the role of those with technical and scientific knowledge as potential enablers and advocates as well as clinicians.

Until recently models of primary health care have been quite hard to find apart from the celebrated example of the Peckham Pioneer Health Centre in South London in the 1930s, which has spawned a strand of succession under the rubric of community-orientated primary care which spread via Johannesburg to Jerusalem and beyond through the work of Sidney Kark and his colleagues. Components of such a system in action could be found with the work of Julian Tudor Hart in South Wales from the 1960s and 1970s as described in his book *A New Kind of Doctor*. The Healthy Living Centre initiative launched by Minister of Public Health Tessa Jowell in 1998 was a short-lived attempt at reorientation which failed to survive a change of government, the same fate being largely met by Sure Start Centres, an evidence-based approach to providing parenting support to families from disadvantaged backgrounds.

A recent example of an imaginative approach to a modern challenge to health and social care can be found in the work of Liverpool family doctor George Kuruvilla in the urban village of Woolton, now home to a rapidly ageing population of professionals, many of whom are bereaved professionals. In 2013 George approached Public Health Director Maggi Morris and myself for help with the increasing issue of lonely older people seeking medical help for a social problem. The way George described it, his waiting room was often full of lonely patients waiting for a chat and a prescription for antidepressants. He was sure that there must be an alternative. Four years later an asset-based approach under the rubric of 'Woolton Community Life—bringing people together' has acquired traction and momentum. With some input from ourselves and John McKnight, George has produced a village directory of a wide range of activities, associations, and clubs available locally. He has established a local community organization with the active support of local traders, faith groups, other community groups, and citizens and recruited dozens of volunteer befrienders. The befrienders take referrals from local family doctors and members of primary care teams and make house visits to familiarize these patients with social options that can help them rediscover the social meaning of life.

Mainstreaming a public health model of primary care runs up against some fundamental obstructions with roots in the lack of a public health orientation to medical education, the failure of universities and professional colleges to embrace interprofessional training, and the short-termism and vicissitudes of government. Professionals who have at the heart of their practice an exclusive focus on the individual patient and their illness struggle to operate in the wider context of social, environmental, and political determinants and the relevance of their own role as community leaders and health advocates. The tribal nature of the organization of the health professions, the domination of institutional models of care, and the subjugation of public health to an individualistic approach to health which denies the importance of collective and government action to protect and improve health, all stand in the way of the holistic and cost-effective approaches to be found in countries such as Finland and Cuba.

The contribution of evidence-based and population-based health care

The application of scientific evidence to population health care as one branch of public health practice has the potential to offer rationality in place of custom and practice and at the same time address issues of allocative efficiency and inequality. With notable exceptions this remains a neglected area of practice with a lack of investment in the skill sets of clinicians that would equip them to play a collaborative leadership role together with public health colleagues.

One example of an attempt to rectify this gap involved Professor Geoffrey Rose of the London School of Hygiene and Tropical Medicine and Professor Kerr White of Johns Hopkins School of Public Health in Baltimore in the 1980s with Kellogg Foundation funding. Hospital physicians were taken out of their workplaces to study epidemiology for 12 months and then returned to clinical practice to apply a population perspective. In the North East of England, Regional Director of Public Health Liam Donaldson allocated public health consultants to work at a number of the region's hospitals, whilst on a lesser scale I managed to place two in the North West. It is salutary to consider how many of the major clinical service failures in recent years might have been avoided if epidemiological expertise had been readily available at top tables to plan, monitor, and surveil services, flagging up outlying outcomes.

One of the leading commentators on the potential for public health input into population health care has been Oxford's Muir Gray, who has approached the matter with evangelical zeal. In seeing population medicine as a new responsibility for the twenty-first century, Gray has identified seven responsibilities (see Table 6.1).

Former Deputy Chief Medical Officer for England Sheila Adam developed pioneering work with the production of epidemiologically based National Service Frameworks to guide the planning and provision of health services in relation to particular conditions and Nick Black of the London School of Hygiene and Tropical Medicine built on earlier work by Walter Holland in the

Table 6.1 Discharging new responsibilities for improving population health in the twenty-first century

New responsibility	Action
Value	Getting the right patients to the right resources
Outcomes	Getting the right outcomes for the right patients
Waste	Getting the right outcomes with the least waste
Sustainability	Doing the right things to protect resources for future generations
Equity	Ensuring fairness and justice
Supporting all patients, not just those referred	Creating population-based integrated systems
Health promotion	Preventing disease and promoting health and wellbeing

evaluation of health services using their public health expertise. Martin McKee, also from the London School, has been a public health pioneer in comparative health care and health care systems across Europe and beyond.

That hospitals should be seen as more than temples of disease and treatment lies behind the World Health Organizations programme for Health Promoting Hospitals, a spin-off of the Healthy Cities Project in which hospitals are seen as resources for health promotion for the communities they serve. A framework for considering specific settings from a public health perspective identified five parameters in the work on healthy prisons (see Box 6.3).

One example of the value of public health research to guide the organization of hospital and health service work is the insights offered from an understanding of environmental conditions on health services. Work by the North West Public Health Observatory has drawn attention to the impact of differing weather conditions on the patterns of sickness and demand which have implications for health service planning and workload. Such an approach can be seen as especially relevant when represented in the form of a calendar of prevalence by medical condition set against the months and seasons.

As this thinking develops there is an evolving curriculum for building capacity and capability in the deployment of epidemiological and other scientific methods in support of population medicine and health care. In his book *Evidence for Population Health*, Dick Heller describes the parameters of this work as including different aspects of the measurement of interventions on

---

Box 6.3 Parameters of a Public Health Framework for Healthy Settings

1. The personal health characteristics of the different demographic groups who inhabit and pass through the setting.
2. Health aspects of the built environment.
3. Health aspects of the natural and surrounding environment.
4. The medical conditions specific to the setting.
5. The relationship of the setting to its environment and surrounding populations as an asset and a resource.

---

health impacts and risks, appropriate outcome measures, the role of health informatics, the management of knowledge, the application of evidence, and questions of priority setting.

Health care needs assessment—contraception, induced abortion, and fertility services

An early example of a systematic approach to a health care needs assessment came from the work in Liverpool on teenage pregnancy. Set against a contextual background and statement of prevalence and incidence data, the framework provided a methodology for systematically exploring the key dimensions to inform service planning and commissioning (see Box 6.4).

Providing a high-quality diabetic retinopathy screening service. The example of Gibraltar

A spell working in Gibraltar provided an opportunity to use epidemiological and public health skills to review the services provided for diabetic retinopathy screening. With a population of only 33,000, Gibraltar represents a relatively small population for whom to provide a diabetic retinopathy screening programme. However, with high smoking, obesity, and type 2 diabetes levels, the need for such services might be anticipated to be greater than many similar-sized communities. With a government health department ambitious to do the best for its population, there were difficult questions to be answered to provide optimal care within limited resources.

> ## Box 6.4 The elements of health needs assessment for contraception, induced abortion, and fertility
>
> 1. Services available and costs
>   - Contraception
>   - Induced abortion
>   - Fertility
> 2. Effectiveness of interventions
> 3. Models of care/recommendation
> 4. Outcome measures, audit, and targets
> 5. Information and research requirements

The prerequisites of a high-quality screening and treatment service are as follows:

- The identification of all known diabetics over the age of 12 years using a diabetic register as a dynamic tool for registration, reminder and recall, and follow-up after treatment;
- A system of digital imaging which is accessible to all patients who should be screened, using up-to-date equipment and software, with standards that are guaranteed through quality assurance and routine clinical audit and external review;
- The export of digital images to a central grading centre, which is operating at scale in order to optimize the conditions for optimal quality control, effectiveness, and efficiency;
- Referral of all patients with unsatisfactory digital images to an optometry and ophthalmology treatment centre for second opinion where necessary and evidence-based, and where quality-assured clinical treatment is available; and
- Follow-up of all patients requiring treatment and pursuit of missing patients who have been called for screening and failed to attend.

In reviewing the local service it was necessary to identify how it was performing against key performance indicators and national (UK) standards, what progress was being made with self-assessment, the viability of the programme size, the availability of high-quality image grading, local clinical governance arrangements and adherence to an integrated common pathway, the robustness of the quality assurance, the integration of the components of the programme, the extent to which the programme was integrated into the wider diabetes agenda, and the extent to which there was meaningful patient feedback.

The outcome was a series of recommendations concerning the optimal screening interval, arrangements for programme management and implementation, the importance of prevention and public health measures, and the shared ownership of the issue.

Whole system public health—the Cumbria journey

In 2006, I moved from working at the North West regional level to the County of Cumbria adjacent to the Scottish border within the North West Region. After 13 years and several radical structural re-organizations of the NHS, I felt it was time for a change. The opportunity presented itself of working in a highly experienced team dealing with a failing system and to undertake fundamental redesign.

Cumbria, as a rural county remote from major urban centres, faced particular challenges in meeting the population health needs of its population within the resources available. It was the third largest county in England in land area, but with a population of only 500,000 spread thinly across a small number of larger towns with most of the population living in small market towns and villages. Shaped like a doughnut sitting on an island, with the famous lakes of the English Lake District at its centre surrounded by mountains, most of the population lived on the periphery. With the exception of the M6 motorway and the West Coast Main Line railway running north to south, transport communications were poor. This was especially a problem on the western side of the county adjacent to the Irish Sea with a ribbon of old industrial settlements characterized by high levels of unemployment and sociomedical stress. In a kaleidoscope of demographics, population groups included hill farmers who struggled to make a living farming sheep in the picturesque uplands, a famous tourist industry characterized by luxury country house hotels but low wages, and relatively affluent outsiders who had chosen to live with the beauty of the area in retirement but in doing so had pushed house prices out of reach of local Cumbrians in an otherwise low-wage economy. The birth rate was low and the population structure rapidly ageing with increasing numbers of frail elderly people often living in isolated poor standard housing with poor access to public services and a shortage of care workers.

The approach we adopted in the NHS Primary Care Trust was based on a philosophy of 'closer to home'. Led by Chief Executive Sue Page, who had a track record of turnaround in health services, and whose motto was 'In God we trust, everybody else must bring data', we set off down a path of evidence-based transformational change. On the executive board the medical director function was shared between a family doctor, a hospital consultant, a community paediatrician, and myself as Director of Public Health jointly appointed with the county council. Sue's first step was to visit all the primary care centres and identify those family doctors with both the passion and skills to lead the transformation to a primary care-led system. My responsibility was to provide the epidemiological and evidence-based underpinning to the necessary changes, to develop the partnerships for health at a whole system level, and to represent the public health-based vision to the Cumbrian community.

Sue's bold step in explicitly promoting primary care leadership through a group of high-performing and committed family doctors had an immediate effect on our way of working, not least for myself. For many years I had tried to engage general practitioners in taking a public health perspective with variable success. In the new situation where they were to lead service developments, the obstacle to this group of doctors taking a population perspective evaporated almost overnight. If they held the responsibility for the whole budget for the whole population, the tension between individual and population levels of intervention was one they would need to grapple with explicitly. At the same time that new responsibility brought with it a growing recognition of the need for whole systems partnership working with local authorities, other public sector organizations, and community organizations and groups. In an environment of constrained resources the recognition that the assets of local people were an important part of the answer became clear.

The role of all of us as Primary Care Trust Directors on this new journey was to position ourselves alongside the general practitioner leadership in a supportive and sometimes coaching style of working, a style akin to community development. We had to start from where the lead clinicians where in their clinical practise and support them in achieving their goals. En route it was necessary to address potentially difficult issues such as potential conflicts of interest; which were met in part by creating a clinical senate as a policy forum with checks and balances. By accepting the responsibility of leadership, the group became aware of its obligations to reconcile individual with group claims on resources and became ever more interested in both a whole population approach and the imperative of work with a range of partners to refocus upstream towards prevention.

I may have had my own agenda for transformational change that included a stress on the importance of health literacy and self-care, place-based working together with the lessons from Peckham and other pioneering efforts. However,

I was able to support and reinforce this reorientation by bringing in resource people of significant experience to share it with them on the basis that 'prophets are never recognized in their own country'. Bringing Lowell Levin from Yale to explore the importance of lay care, John McKnight from Illinois on asset-based community development, and Leon Epstein from Jerusalem to share his experience of community-orientated primary care with a multidisciplinary audience of public and voluntary sector Cumbria leadership could have much more impact than the local DPH telling them what to do! Refreshing too was a willingness of our board to support fact-finding trips to North America and Finland to witness different approaches to population health care at first hand with the side benefit that I was able to send my health protection consultant to Copenhagen to become acquainted with the Danish forensic approach to eliminating hospital-acquired infection.

My link in holding a joint appointment with the county council initially began to pay dividends too. The chief executive at the council, Peter Stybelski, was a highly intelligent and creative man who welcomed my arrival as somebody who would bring in challenging and new ideas. Sadly, the county had a history of poor public services with weak leadership, characterized by a paternalistic approach, symptomatic of a lingering feudal past. In addition it was ludicrously over-administered with three layers of government comprising a county, six districts, dozens of parish councils, and literally over 1000 councillors, all of which introduced fragmentations of function, petty jealousies, and turf wars. Until his early retirement because of ill health, Chief Executive Peter Stybelski was able to overcome much of this with his vision, charm, and humanity. After he had gone, Cumbria was not so fortunate but a legacy was the production of the first whole county strategy for health and wellbeing. This strategy identified the scope for joint working on health inequalities and for mobilizing community resources to tackle the related challenges of physical fitness levels, obesity, tobacco, excess alcohol consumption, sexual health, and mental health and wellbeing. By the time I left Cumbria in 2013 the modestly sized public health team had created an influential presence both at the county level and in the district councils, especially with their responsibilities for housing, environmental health, and community development. At the same time the city of Carlisle, a small player among cities, demonstrated its ambition by successfully applying to become part of the WHO European Healthy City network.

Intelligence

The earlier experience of working in Liverpool and across the North West had underlined the importance of good public health intelligence in creating the momentum for innovation and change. The starting point in Cumbria was to produce the first whole county public health report, published in 2008 together with a widely distributed booklet and DVD based on a public lecture which had identified five challenges for the county (Box 6.5).

Box 6.5 Five challenges for public health in Cumbria

1. The demographic challenge

With one in five Cumbrian women childless into their forties and a projected large increase in those living beyond 85, with the numbers of those with dementia estimated to increase from 6,000 to 10,000 over the next 20 years, the county faces a double whammy in the near future. For every three people newly retiring for only two leaving school there would be a major labour shortage for entry into the caring professions at the very time that need and demand would be increasing. A fully engaged and asset-based approach to care was going to be critical.

2. Inequalities in health and levelling up

The public health report revealed a massive 17-year difference in life expectancy between the most and least disadvantaged wards in the county. Quite apart from the social injustice of this, it was a drag on the local economy, with high levels of sickness absence and a burden of care which simultaneously increased the demand on health and social services and reduced the available human resource for the workforce.

3. Reorientation health and social care services to be closer to home

The pattern of health and disease in the county, together with the demographic and economic position, pointed to a dysfunctional distribution with the wrong kind of services located in suboptimal locations for quality, access, and efficiency of resource allocation. A transformation to a primary care-led service with full public engagement and strong primary and community care was the only solution with a prospect of meeting the competing demands.

4. A health system based on intelligence

Sue Page's mantra 'In God we Trust, everybody else must bring data' was music to a public health director's ears. At last here was an opportunity for

Box 6.5 Five challenges for public health in Cumbria *(continued)*

evidence-based intelligence of cause and effect, intervention, and outcome to take its place alongside the director of finance reports at commissioning and board meetings. These first reports were followed up by a series of lifecycle-based reports commissioned from the North West Public Health Observatory which covered birth to old age and death.

The Cumbria Lifecycle Reports

1. Born in Cumbria

2. Coming of Age in Cumbria

3. Living Well in Cumbria

4. Growing Older in Cumbria

5. Mortality in Cumbria.

In addition a pocket-sized booklet, 'Cumbria in Numbers', combining practical vital, demographic, and health statistics down to a local government ward level was produced to enable local politicians and interested others to have the data, most meaningful to them, at their fingertips.

A policy of producing these public health reports in A5 book size was adopted. This enabled readers to keep them with other books on their shelves and extended their use and accessibility. The 2012 report, which included a personal resilience guide for emergency preparedness, won the national prize for the best public health report of the year; the 2013 report threw the spotlight on the topical issue of the health and wellbeing of military veterans in the aftermath of conflicts in the gulf states—'Those Who Have Served'; and a special report was commissioned from the North West Observatory on health aspects of the nuclear industry.

5. Building capacity

The publication of Sir Derek Wanless' 'Fully Engaged Scenario' had significant implications for the challenge of whole systems engagement and citizen involvement in the co-production and protection of health. The implementation of this transformation had implied that maintaining health is a partnership at every level—for individuals, within neighbourhoods and communities, within and between employers and other agencies, and within local, national, and international government and regulatory bodies. It implied a transformation of the relationship between citizens and professionals and bureaucracies. In Cumbria we pursued these goals by adopting an Investment for Health approach, making explicit the total resources available across the public sector for health and wellbeing and by deploying the

Box 6.5 Five challenges for public health in Cumbria *(continued)*

public health professionals in a matrix fashion across the county. The asset-based approach to community development was promoted together with extensive settings based work on Healthy Schools and Healthy Cities and support for a community-orientated approach to primary care. A Cumbria Health Observatory was established in the county council, drawing on the experience of the Liverpool Observatories.

Clinical governance and the Tuesday 'ward rounds'—the bonding impact of serious untoward Incidents

Having worked at a regional and national level and having had experience of major incidents at a community level turned out to be a good background for the succession of events that hit Cumbria from 2007 onwards. A rail crash, floods, school bus tragedy, SARS, swine flu, and a mass shooting incident, all tested our systems and helped forge good interagency arrangements. The one exception would turn out to be the safeguarding of the county's children.

My experience as Regional Medical Officer had included working alongside the new breed of clinical and medical directors in hospital trusts in the 1990s to help them develop their role. In addition my responsibility for following up doctors who were in trouble with the General Medical Council for poor performance stood me in good stead when it came to the shared work of medical director in the Primary Care Trust. I also had the unusual experience of being Regional Medical Officer at the time when one of the North West's family doctors, Harold Shipman, was exposed as a mass murderer of his patients. In March 1998, a colleague of Shipman's had expressed concern to the local coroner about the large numbers of deaths occurring among Shipman's patients. It would be some months before police investigation would reveal that he had killed an estimated 250 people, mostly women. Although not directly involved in the investigation I was subsequently required to follow up on questionable prescribing practices that were revealed by the police poring over doctors' pharmacy records. This led to uncomfortable scrutiny of some clinical practice, a reminder, as in the aftermath of BSE, that audit trails of decisions made and actions pursued can have legal repercussions. When the dust settled, a statistical analysis of deaths in the Shipman practice found a massive excess of observed over expected numbers of deaths, something that in the current state of primary care record-keeping would not be revealed by routine monitoring.

As the Primary Care Trust of Medical Directors bedded in, we began to suspect that although routine data tended to indicate that by and large Cumbria was generally average for measures of population health and clinical outcomes, these averages may hide services that were not as good as they should be given the population's demographics. We were concerned that the groundbreaking work by Chief Medical officer Liam Donaldson in his report 'Organization with a Memory' was not being followed through. The work sought to import the lessons of the airline industry about transparency, learning from near misses and creating a no-blame, learning culture. A spate of sporadic reports of untoward events, not least with regard to maternal and child health and suicide among mental health patients, caused us to take stock and explore ways of putting our oversight on a more systematic basis. The upshot was to establish a regular weekly virtual, 'ward round', involving all our own medical directors, which would receive and review clinical incidents that had been drawn to our attention and to develop systematic visits and discussions with hospital clinical and medical directors as a developmental process. A third strand of the approach was to have regular meetings with those responsible for clinical quality. The value of this was to become evident when a number of serious clinical incidents came to light.

Our efforts to professionalize the performance management of clinical failure and near misses were hampered by the ambiguity of responsibility that had recently emerged following the abolition of the Regional Health Authority and its replacement by a Strategic Health Authority that seemed more focused on satisfying health ministers in London than looking out for patients on the ground. Our antennae were alerted by incidents where there appeared to have been poor clinical input, for example with regard to the availability of medical consultants at nights and weekends to support junior colleagues, by clinical incidents that we came to hear about but had not been notified of, by the tardiness of reporting other serious events, and by a general sense that the system was not committed to reflection and learning. There were issues too with regard to overlapping responsibilities when patients were in the care of more than one organization, as for example when a psychiatric patient was admitted to a general medical unit and took their own life. We were concerned with how the intelligence derived from the reporting of all deaths of Cumbrians under the age of 18 years to the under 18 death panel were being handled and with a steady stream of serious untoward incidents involving the death or injury of children which appeared to show that lessons were not being learned. The children's safeguarding agenda was regularly being subject to criticism by external watchdogs but little seemed to change. In engaging with this agenda we also found that there had been a failure to ensure that all health service staff had undertaken training in child protection and safeguarding, something that was within our powers to rectify and we did.

Safeguarding—it takes a village to protect the vulnerable

The safeguarding of vulnerable children and adults has been a prominent issue for many years in the United Kingdom with regular reports of a child being killed or seriously harmed by those who are responsible for their care. The fate of older people, perhaps with dementia, whose fragility can make them particularly helpless, especially in badly run care homes, is no less of a scandal. In my time in Cumbria we had to deal with a number of the former but fortunately less of the latter; in addition one young girl had been groomed for sexual exploitation by the staff of a food-take-away shop.

Each time a serious case review was initiated I was shocked, not only at the failure to learn the lessons from the previous one but also by the narrow approach taken, with an over-dependence on the intervention of professionals to deal with a community problem. John McKnight's mantra that 'it takes a village (neighbourhood or community) to raise a child' is not only true of children, but also of the protection of other vulnerable and underserved groups. There will never be enough social workers to guarantee the safety of all the children at risk, just as there will never be enough social media staff to protect the two billion Internet users against obscene or dangerous content. The steady professionalization and fragmentation of the organized efforts of society in recent years had been accompanied by societal changes that, together, put children at greater risk. This had not been helped by a media-generated moral panic about paedophilia which had been counterproductive in generating a climate where adults were reluctant to show any interest in the welfare of other people's children for fear of being misconstrued. The jealously guarded silos and fiefdoms that had replaced the public health departments of old had served to consolidate the dysfunction with a result that each time a child was harmed, the response seemed to be to put in place a further round of performance management box ticking designed to protect the backs of senior managers with an increasingly demoralized front-line staff.

An example of the untoward consequences of these trends can be illustrated by an incident I was involved with on one of my work trips to London. Returning from Euston station to catch the last evening train north, I came across a young girl aged 14 or 15 in distress at the ticket barrier. Having been to London for the day she had lost her ticket home and had no more money, and the rail official refused to let her board the train. She was faced with being stranded overnight in London with all its hazards and risks for a young person. It brought to mind a meeting I had had some years previously with the Governor of Visakhapatnam on the eastern seaboard of India. He told me that each evening when he had finished the day's work he would go with his driver in the official car to the main station. Here he would round up all the newly arrived, desperate children and young people, who had travelled from around the state during the day, and take them to a place of safety. I paid the young girl's fare and she was able to get home.

The problem of young people running away from home, and frequently abuse, to the big cities, is common in most countries; many young people from the North of England finish up in London where fate may hold dreadful futures for them. At the next meeting of the senior officers in the council I made a suggestion that perhaps we could take space in 'The Big Issue', a newspaper sold by homeless people, to help them into the world of work and give them some income. Perhaps we could provide a contact number for northern youngsters to phone if they wanted to come back to their home area with a train ticket paid for, and the guarantee that their wishes with regard to future contact with their families would be respected. To say that my proposal fell on stony ground is an understatement.

I see safeguarding primarily as a public health issue that requires a whole system response and a change of culture from a bureaucratic one to a proactive one. It is no coincidence that the governor of Visakhapatnam and my old friend Slobodan Lang shared the same approach to making themselves accessible to the people who they served. At the end of each day in Visag, the governor would be publicly available for an hour to be petitioned about matters that concerned them. In Zagreb, Slobodan took the same approach on health matters once a month. Soviet dictator Joseph Stalin asked how many troops the Pope had. The troops for protection of the vulnerable are ordinary citizens who accept that in the most appropriate way they are their brothers' and sisters' and children's keepers. Our role is to support active citizenship with knowledge, skills, signposting, and professional support. It is an asset-based approach.

Underserved groups

The population approach at the heart of public health works with three types of population: the whole population; populations at risk; and populations that have defined conditions. Cutting across these are what the World Health Organization calls underserved groups, who, by virtue of their special circumstances may fall between the gaps of the system. Such groups might include refugees, the homeless, children in or leaving the care of local authorities, sex workers, prisoners, their partners and families, or military veterans returned from conflict. At the very local level their numbers may be too small to register on anybody's radar, whereas at the district or regional level they may constitute a large enough statistical group to think about strategically. Bearing in mind the refection by the late Major Greenwood of the London School of Hygiene and Tropical Medicine that 'Statistics are people with the tears wiped off', our shared task is to understand the statistics and then to put in place humane service responses.

The role of the media—taking people on a journey

It is not so long ago that health care organizations saw public engagement and media relations as very much a second-order activity that was often left to a junior member of staff. Among the first National Health Service organizations to realize the value of investing in good health communications was the West Midlands and also Wessex where I had cut my public health teeth in the 1970s. In Birmingham, pioneering Regional Medical Officer Rod Griffiths and his media lead Paul Castle had managed to make real progress with fluoridating the water supplies through intelligent engagement with the general public, before the forces of irrationality were galvanized and such moves became all but impossible elsewhere. In Wessex, where I was struggling with the politics of abortion, Ian Dillow, with a professional background in journalism, was able to school me and colleagues in the basic arts of crafting succinct messages and making them count.

It was, however, under Sir Donald Wilson in Liverpool in the mid-1980s that I first had the opportunity of being a part of a systematic approach to health communication that raised things to another level. Sir Donald's enthusiastic embrace of our health promotion activities at the International Garden Festival in 1984 led him to sanction support for the secondment, part time, of a dynamic young worker from the largest public relations agency on Merseyside. Almost immediately we began to achieve massive, virtually free coverage in live and print media for public health and disease prevention. From being a passive and reactive activity the potential for making the weather rather than responding to it became obvious. The next phase in the development of this essential strand of our work in the North West came with the recruitment of journalist and local radio broadcaster Hugh Lamont, who proceeded to put it on a robust and regular footing, exploiting the newly emerging tools such as video to engage with local people by using people, places, and issues that they could identify with. Years later Baroness Julia Cumberlege, former Minister for Health whom I had worked closely with, reminded me how powerful had been a video we had made on the issues behind her 'Changing Childbirth' initiative in creating momentum by giving voice to local pregnant women. By the time I arrived in Cumbria in 2006, I was clear of the importance of having systematic health communications if we were to have any impact with the 'closer to home' agenda and the transformation of the Cumbrian system. Fortunately, this view was shared by all my colleagues who brought with them their own positive experiences of active media engagement.

Between 2006 and 2013, the Cumbrian Primary Care Trust consistently punched above its own weight in health communications. Under the leadership of two highly experienced experts in change management, crafted messages, and the dark arts of politics, Ross Forbes and Mark Graham put this activity on a professional and systematic basis. In a previous life Mark had been assistant to a member of parliament and government minister and he imported to our small organization the practical mechanism of a communications grid. Each week by Friday afternoon we had a clear plan of action for making the weather the following week, whether it was setting the agenda in support of our own transformational ambitions, the actions and progress on the implications of our public health intelligence work, or responding to the latest left-field incident impacting on public health. Month after month throughout these years external monitoring and evaluation of media coverage documented how Cumbria achieved more reporting and more positive reporting than any other health organization in the North West region. It was a pity then that some of the other health organizations that were coming under pressure with adverse incidents continued in a reactive and defensive mode instead of embracing collaboration with the media and others that could be of such help.

When things go wrong

Organ retention at the Royal Liverpool Children's Hospital—the Alder Hey

In September 1999, it emerged that the organs of large numbers of deceased infants and children from the Alder Hey Children's Hospital in Liverpool had been retained for 'research purposes' by clinicians without their parents' consent. Subsequent events would send shock waves across the country and beyond, would end careers, change medical practice, and raise fundamental questions about the ethical underpinnings of professional governance. They would also reveal serious shortcomings in the way that health organizations handled serious untoward incidents in the media and led to a crisis of confidence by the public in their professional advisers. One of the depressing things is that it didn't have to be that way.

Spending many years observing Sir Donald Wilson at work as a health authority chairman, the message was always clear. In large, complex organizations, providing medical care to millions of people, things will sometimes go wrong. We have a responsibility to strive for the highest standards and to minimize harm but when things go wrong the rules are simple:

1. You put your hands up and admit it, and apologize (properly).
2. You take immediate steps to ascertain the full facts and share them in a spirit of transparency.
3. You learn the lessons across the organization and do everything to prevent a recurrence.

If you don't follow these rules you let everybody down, cause immense damage, not least to those affected and their loved ones, and at the same time cause immense damage to the organization that you might be trying to protect. If you are intransigent and insensitive, careers may well end and heads roll as they did in the case of Alder Hey.

So what had happened at Alder Hey? In a nutshell there had been for many years a widespread practice internationally of pathologists retaining organs and tissue samples for research and teaching. This had often been without either formal consent or clear objectives of intent for their use or proper subsequent disposal. In the case of the Liverpool pathologist Professor van Velzen, the retention of organs took on a grotesque life of its own. His failures to organize his workload led to a backlog of large numbers of organs and specimens which I personally witnessed in a storeroom in the University of Liverpool. Row upon row of plastic paint pots on shelves in a semi-basement containing the tissues of children; tissues which parents believed had been included in ritual funeral arrangements for burial or cremation as part of the grieving process. The collection included 1,564 stillbirths or pre-viable foetuses, 188 eyes, whole bodies, a separated head, and a large number of brains. The reason given for keeping the families in the dark was the paternalistic one that it was supposedly in their best interests and those of future patients by reducing the mortality rate of surgery for congenital cardiac malformations, something that the later official inquiry rejected.

The scandal surrounding the revelations at Alder Hey rumbled on for over three years and is still having an effect many years later. The situation was very badly handled by the hospital and its management team who initially failed to accept the enormity of what had happened and generally failed to recognize the sensitivity and hurt that had been caused. Blame fell not only on the hospital but on the university that employed some of the clinical staff, with the governance arrangements being particularly singled out. Professor van Velzen and the hospital chief executive left their jobs and the affair had an impact on the practice of pathology and the functioning of coroners. One unanticipated consequence of the hospital coming under intense scrutiny was to put the outcomes for paediatric cardiac surgery into the spotlight, with families expressing concern at varying outcomes depending on the surgeon operating. As a result Health Minister Philip Hunt asked me to review the outcome data, which I did with the support of my statistical analyst Tom Hennell. This exercise threw into relief not only the methodological challenge of evaluating outcomes with small numbers, but also the conundrum that in highly specialized clinical practice where there may a small number of skilled clinicians, it is impossible for all patients to be treated by the one with apparently the best results. As a result of my report the minister was able to make progress with the goal of putting into the public domain clinicians' outcome data.

The Alder Hey episode as a disaster—the recovery phase

My own interest in what happened at Alder Hey extended beyond the professional to the personal. My older sister had given birth to a child in the 1960s in Liverpool, with congenital cardiac abnormalities. She survived for only a day or two and was taken away from her mother to be disposed of, without a funeral or place to remember her. I was reminded of this on a visit to the cemetery island of San Michele in Venice where there is a special area for the burial of the children. Following events at the Alder Hey I had discussions with the new chairman and management team and with the Bishop of Liverpool about how the hospital and its community could heal. One way of publicly recognizing the importance of responding to the emotional needs of bereaved parents was to be a special garden in the grounds of the new hospital that was just being planned. More strategically it was accepted that the adoption of a systematic approach to hospital arts could be a vehicle for cultural transformation. It has been a great source of satisfaction to see how this important Liverpool institution has developed its programme of artistic activities in their many forms over the ensuing years.

The failure of a breast screening programme in a Cumbrian hospital

In the spring of 2010, the lead for breast screening quality assurance in the North West contacted me to share her concerns about the breast screening service provided to the women of North Cumbria from the Cumberland Infirmary in Carlisle. Monitoring of the service had shown that it was failing to detect the expected number of breast cancer cases as would be expected in a population of its size. As Director of Public Health I called a major incident and convened an incident group meeting at the hospital. An independent review of 1,600 breast screening patient records spanning the previous three years was commissioned which identified that 100–150 women of the 45,000 women screened during that period would require further investigation involving biopsy. Eventually 16 women were identified who had been told that their breasts were healthy when in fact they had breast cancer which should have led to treatment. I had no alternative but to suspend the service and find an alternative immediate provider with a different service in the longer term.

It transpired that the underlying issues concerned poor clinical governance of the service with a failure to adhere to up-to-date clinical protocols and carry out needle biopsies on those women where it was indicated. The initial response of the hospital and its clinicians was defensive with a reluctance to recognize the seriousness of the problem, preferring to represent it as a communication issue between the hospital and other agencies. The patients affected were angry and disillusioned with the National Health Service locally and especially critical of the way they had been communicated with. Although it appears that our prompt intervention meant that no lives were lost, the episode resulted in severe reputational damage to the hospital and trust in its clinical services together with effective legal action by three of the patients.

The scandal at Morecambe Bay University Hospitals Trust—a slow burn corporate clinical disaster

Morecambe Bay University Hospitals Trust consists of three hospitals that between them provide secondary and some tertiary medical care for 350,000 people living around the estuary of the River Lune and Morecambe Bay. Three hospitals had been brought together as one organization, Lancaster Royal Infirmary being the largest and most comprehensive as well as the most prestigious in view of its teaching hospital status with alignment to the highly regarded University of Lancaster. Although regarded as a district general hospital in its own right, a smaller hospital at Barrow-in-Furness, serving a population of under 100,000, struggled to recruit staff and to offer a full range of secondary care clinical services. The third hospital at Kendal was widely regarded to have been built as a political manoeuvre to protect the parliamentary seat of the sitting member of parliament and from the beginning, it had experienced a trimming back of the range of services it provided, a particularly contentious issue having been the withdrawal of its coronary care unit.

My exposure to Morecambe Bay began with my first visit to establish contact with the medical director in the spring of 2007. My first impression was one of surprise to find that such a key person as the medical director was in an office that was not only not close to that of the chief executive but on a different floor.

I received a warm response from somebody who seemed very committed to his job but was put on the alert during the course of our conversation to hear that he had only just been informed about a perinatal death in the Barrow maternity unit that had occurred some months before. My concerns were raised about the system for notifying potentially serious clinical incidents and this was reinforced the following week when I was contacted to tell me of a second historic perinatal death.

This was early in the existence of the new Primary Care Trust for Cumbria and I was in the process of researching my first public health report. This was showing unremarkable maternal and infant mortality statistics with no evidence of any outliers compared with the regional or national position. However, I had become sensitized to the issue and there were to be straws in the wind that such statistical monitoring may not be telling the whole story; over the next few years there were three maternal deaths at Barrow, two in one year and one the next, compared to the several dozen maternal deaths occurring nationally in a population of 60 million. This might have been expected to have prompted concern and enhanced clinical audit, especially when all three women had been born overseas.

Other data which I scrutinized at this time and which began to reinforce my anxieties revealed big differences in clinical practice between the hospitals with regard to hysterectomy and episiotomy operation rates and it also became clear that it was very difficult for Barrow women to obtain a termination of pregnancy at their local hospital. On enquiry other issues began to provide soft evidence of a poorly governed and functioning triple-headed hospital. For example, the challenge of multisite hospital working had never been properly addressed by putting in place multisite hospital consultant contracts to facilitate movement and mutual support between the three hospitals. In turn this had contributed to difficulties in recruitment outside of the university city of Lancaster. My concerns were reinforced on a visit to the Lancaster Infirmary with a friend who was attending for clinical assessment of his newly diagnosed cancer to find medical records strewn around the outpatient department in piles. One of the emerging problems following the 2006 National Health Service reorganization was yet one more major disruption to interorganizational arrangements, leading to confusion of managerial responsibilities. This was to prove important as events unfolded.

By 2010, my concerns were such that I decided that it was time to look into matters in greater detail and commissioned an in-depth analysis from the North West Public Health Observatory whilst simultaneously looking for a team to carry out a robust external review of perinatal mortality. Having access to the observatory with its team of analysts who were accustomed to turning round high-quality reports in a reasonable timescale was one thing; tracking down an experienced multidisciplinary perinatal clinical audit team when government funding had recently been withdrawn from the leading unit at Oxford was something else. By the time the work could be undertaken it had been largely overtaken by events.

In November 2008, baby Joshua Titcombe died from pneumococcal septicaemia and pulmonary haemorrhage nine days after his birth in the maternity unit in Barrow-in Furness. He had been transferred to Manchester where he died and as a result his death did not show up in the Barrow statistics. Joshua's father, James Titcombe, was a project manager in the nuclear industry at Cumbria's Sellafield power station with a profound knowledge of safety systems in complex organizations. Following Joshua's death, James embarked on a long campaign to expose the failings of clinical care and governance and do justice to his dead son, to the family, and to the community served by the three Morecambe Bay hospitals.

It took from 2009 when James Titcombe made a complaint to the Health Service Ombudsman until 2012 when an NHS Gold Command was called by the North West Strategic Health Authority at the instigation of myself and the Cumbria Primary Care Trust,[1] before the wheels were set in motion to deal with a whole systems failure and clinical scandal. Subsequently the inquiry chaired by Dr Bill Kirkup[2] revealed that there had been systemic clinical failures at the hospitals characterized by a dysfunctional maternity unit, delayed problem recognition with missed opportunities to recognize them, together with a cluster of five serious incidents in 2008 involving one maternal and three perinatal deaths and an infant who sustained serious damage. The response of the Hospitals Trust had been defensive to the extent of keeping confidential a report it had commissioned into its maternity care by Dame Pauline Fielding, in August 2010, which had included significant criticisms of maternity care, including dysfunctional relationships, poor environment, and a poor approach to clinical governance and effectiveness. It had apparently been held back from

---

[1] The Medical Directors of Cumbria Primary Care Trust: Mike Bewick, Neela Shabde, Irving Cobden, John Ashton. County Nursing Director Moira Angel.

[2] Bill Kirkup, former Regional Director of Public Health in the North East of England and former Deputy Chief Medical Officer to Sir Liam Donaldson. Not for the first time did Bill put his public health skills to good use in the cause of righting an injustice. As a member of Liverpool's Bishop James Jones Hillsborough Disaster Review Panel, Bill systematically reviewed the clinical and pathological post mortem data with clinical colleagues and concluded that many of those who died at Hillsborough might have had a chance of surviving if the emergency response had functioned properly.

wider circulation for fear that it could impede the hospitals attaining founda-
tion trust status and was not shared with the Strategic Health Authority until
October 2010 and with the external bodies, the Care Quality Commission, and
'Monitor' until April 2011.

The Public Health Observatory statistical review was published in February
2013, once again appearing to show a neutral position but lacking data on patient transfers to tertiary centres. The detailed, qualitative, and much delayed
multidisciplinary review of perinatal deaths was especially revealing in its findings about the use of serious untoward incident reviews and local investigations. Of the 20 cases identified with at least one major avoidable factor, only
one had been reported as a serious untoward incident with four having a review
from case notes. The expert panel assessed the single serious untoward incident
report, finding it to be inadequate and lacking in content and detail on the lessons to be learnt. The report also highlighted the important association of very
high obesity and smoking rates among women whose baby died in the perinatal
period.

When colleagues and I in the Primary Care Trust heard about the Fielding
Report that same spring, I insisted on us setting up regular incident meetings
which were attended by representatives of the Strategic Health Authority. It
was with great reluctance that they agreed to us declaring a major incident,
expressing concern that they had too much on their plate as they were already
dealing with one major incident in Stockport in greater Manchester where a
nurse was suspected of poisoning her patients. The calling of a Gold Command
brought with it the benefit of the NHS outside of the Hospital Trust itself being
able to intervene at a strategic level as a matter of urgency. Unfortunately, this
was delayed as a result of the Strategic Health Authority dragging its feet but
would eventually lead to effective intervention as well as a proper legal inquiry.

Bill Kirkup's report on his investigation reviewed the deaths of more than 200
mothers and babies between 2004 and 2013, concluding that up to 19 infants
and mothers died at the University of Morecambe Bay Hospitals as a result of
poor care. James Titcombe's campaign on behalf of his son was vindicated, dis-
ciplinary action was taken against midwives, careers were ended, and immense
damage was done to the hospitals' reputation and to trust in its clinicians.

Meanwhile some 100 miles south of Lancaster at Stafford Hospital another
health care clinical scandal had been unfolding involving high mortality rates
that had gone unnoticed because of the lack of epidemiological expertise and
public health monitoring and poor clinical governance. Claims were made that
between 400 and 1200 more patients died between 2005 and 2008 than might
have been expected.

Reference

1. **Morris, J. N.** Are health services important to the people's health? *British Medical Journal* **280**(6208) (1980), 167–8.

Further Reading

Abel-Smith, B. *A History of the Nursing Profession.* London: Heinemann, 1960.

Abel-Smith, B. *The Hospitals.* London: Heinemann, 1964.

Ashton, J. Public health and primary care: towards a common agenda. *Public Health* **104** (1990), 387–98.

Ashton, J. R. *Review of the Cardiac Unit at the Royal Liverpool Children's Hospital NHS Trust Alder Hey.* NHS Executive, North west, 2000.

Boston Women's Health Collective. *The New Our Bodies Ourselves.* New York: Simon and Schuster, 1984.

Considerations for Commissioners in NHS Diabetic Eye Screening Procurement. NHS Diabetic Eye Screening Programme, NHS England, 2014.

Cumbria 2011. *The Annual Report of the Director of Public Health.* Cumbria County Council/NHS Cumbria.

Cumbria 2012. *The Annual Report of the Director of Public Health.* Cumbria County Council/NHS Cumbria.

Cumbria County Council/Cumbria Primary Care Trust. *Health in Cumbria 2008: The Annual Report of the Director of Public Health*, 2008.

Cumbria County Council/Cumbria Primary Care Trust. *The Five Challenges: Inaugural Public Health lecture by Professor John R Ashton, CBE* (2008).

Cumbria Intelligence Observatory/Cumbria County Council/ NHS Cumbria. *Cumbria in Numbers* 2013.

Cumbria NHS Primary Care Trust/ Cumbria County Council. *Health and Wellbeing Strategy, 2008-2011* (2008).

Delamothe, T. Using outcomes research. *BMJ 308* (1994), 1583–4.

Department of Health. Healthy Living Centres, report of a seminar. London: Department of Health, 1998.

Department of Health. Report of a Census of Organs and Tissues Retained by Pathology Services in England. Conducted by the Chief Medical Officer. London: HM Stationery Office, 2006.

Diabetic Eye Screening: programme overview. (2014). Public Health England.

Epstein, L., J. Gofin, R. Gofin, and **Y. Neumark.** The Jerusalem experience—three decades of service, research, and training in community-oriented primary care. *American Journal of Public Health* **92**(11) (2002), 1717–21.

Greek, M. D. Serving the cause of public health. Selected Papers of Andria Stampar. Zagreb: Andrijar Stampar School of Public Health, 1966.

Health Care Needs Assessment. *The Epidemiologically Based Needs Assessment Reviews*, first series, second edition, Vol. **2**, edited by **A. Stevens, J. Raftery, J. Mant,** and **S. Simpson.** Oxford: Radcliffe, 2004.

Heller, R. *Evidence for Population Health.* Oxford: Oxford University Press, 2005.

Hughes, S., M. A. Bellis, W. Bird, J. R. Ashton. Weather Forecasting as a Public Health Tool. Centre for Public Health, Liverpool John Moores University, 2004.

Illich, I. *Medical Nemesis—the Expropriation of Health.* London: Marion Boyars, 1975.

Kark, S. L. *The Practice of Community Oriented Primary Health Care.* New York: Appleton-Century-Crofts, 1981.

Kirkup, B. The Report of the Morecambe Bay Investigation. (2015).

Levin, L. S., and E. L. Idler. *The Hidden Health Care System.* Golden Apple, 2010.

Levin, L. S., A. H. Katz, and E. Holst. *Self-Care.* London: Crook Helm, 1977.

McKnight, J. *The Careless Society: Community and its Counterfeits.* New York: Perseus Books, 1995.

McKnight, J., and P. Blok. The Abundant Community: Awakening the Power of Families and Neighbourhoods. San Francisco: American Planning Association and Barrett-Koehler, 2010.

Morris, J. N. Are health services important to the people's health? *British Medical Journal* **280**(6208) (1980), 167–8.

Morris, J. N. *Uses of Epidemiology.* Edinburgh: Churchill Livingstone, 1975.

Muir Gray, J. A. *How to Practise Population Medicine.* Oxford: Offox Press, 2013.

Oakley, A., and Barker J. *Private Complaints and Public Health: Richard Titmuss on the National Health Service.* Bristol: The Policy Press, 2004.

Pearse, I. H., and L. H. Crocker. *The Peckham Experiment: A Study of the Living Structure of Society.* London: Allen and Unwin, 1947.

Public Health Report. *Those Who Have Served.* Cumbria: Cumbria Intelligence Observatory /Cumbria County Council/NHS, 2013–.

Royal Liverpool Children's Inquiry Report. London: HM Stationery Office, 2001.

Titcombe, J. *Joshua's Story: Uncovering the Morecambe Bay Scandal.* Leeds: Anderson Wallace, 2015.

Tudor Hart, J. *A New Kind of Doctor: The General Practitioner's Part in the Health of the Community.* London: Merlin Press, 1988.

Ubido, Janet, Lyn Winters, Matthew Ashton, Alex Scott-Samuel, Janet Atherton, and **Fiona Johnstone.** *Top Tips for Healthier Hospitals.* Liverpool Public Health Observatory and Cheshire and Merseyside Public Health Network, 2006.

Vuori, H. Primary care in industrialised countries. In Die Allgemeinpraxix; Das Zentrum Derek bArtzlichen, pp 83–111. Zurich: Grundverorgung Gottlieb Duttwierer—Institut Ruschlikon, 1981.

Wanless, D. *Securing our Future Health: Taking a Long Term View. The Public Enquiry Unit.* London: HM Treasury, 2002.

Wood, J. *Rural Health and Healthcare. A north west perspective: A Public Health Information Report.* Institute for Health Research Lancaster University/ North West Public Health Observatory, 2004.

Woolton Community Life Directory (2015). Available at http://www. wooltoncommunitylife.org.uk

Part III

Synthesis

Chapter 7

No health without mental health—*mens sana in corpore sano*

In 2016 then Prime Minister Cameron announced a new initiative on mental health with a particular emphasis on parenting classes. It came at a time when there was increasing concern at the state of the nation's mental health with a flurry of documents and reports, a campaign led by *The Times* newspaper, and increased demand for parity of resourcing between mental and physical health. Some of the pressure to do something specifically about child and adolescent mental health was coming from private schools who were witnessing increasing levels of emotional distress among children from affluent backgrounds. This was manifested in the levels of general anxiety and depression, eating disorders, self-harm, and other behavioural disturbances.

Those monitoring the epidemiology of child and adolescent mental health were reporting that the historic estimated levels of morbidity of 5–10 per cent were now being exceeded. That it should be among the more advantaged sectors of the community that were concerned was unusual. Not for the first time a public health issue not confined to the poor was beginning to galvanize community leaders into action; it had been similar in the cholera days and during the HIV/AIDS outbreak. Enlightened self-interest has often been the driver for action on public health threats.

As one who began his early career as a psychiatrist, the increased focus on mental health has a particular poignancy to me. As a medical student my interests spanned the humanities as well as the natural sciences. History and politics were always as interesting to me as biology and when I came across the prospectus for the public health masters course at the London School of Hygiene and Tropical Medicine it was clear to me that sooner or later I would be signing up. For the next 10 years I would religiously send for each new edition of the prospectus. Fortunately, my interest was nurtured and kept alive by the remarkable social orientation of the Newcastle medical course. The school was imbued with the spirit not only of the pioneering community-orientated paediatrician Sir James Spence, but also that of Aberdonian obstetrician Sir Dugald Baird through his Newcastle disciples. The strong social and community base was reinforced by a series of deans of medicine who, while hard-nosed neurologists and endocrinologists themselves, supported the work of those such as John Walker, who integrated teaching in public health and primary care and GP Sir Donald Irvine, who was instrumental in establishing the country's first general practice training programme and later took charge of the General Medical Council. It was under Sir Donald's supervision that I was to become co-author of the first UK publication on clinical audit in general practice.

When I began my psychiatric training I quickly became frustrated at the failure of mental health services to focus upstream to the promotion of mental health and prevention of mental illness. This was at a time in the heady post-sixties era when there was a strong focus on mental health and the controversies created by so-called anti-psychiatrists such as R. D. Laing, Thomas Szasz, and Aaron Estersson. As juniors we were exposed to the whole spectrum of ideas from Freud and Jung to the phenomenologists Kraepelin and Eliot Slater and the organic school of psychiatry associated with people like William Sargent. The Newcastle School itself was grounded in psychiatric epidemiology. Although we had opportunities to cut our teeth on individual, group, and marital therapy, the broader public health agenda remained elusive. I came to the conclusion that what was on offer was too little and too late and as soon as I finished my training I moved into general practice in the hope of finding more fertile soil in prevention.

My next move took me to Southampton, where the pioneering dean of the new medical school, Donald Acheson, had created an exciting opportunity for somebody like myself. In a university-run community health centre, based on lines proposed by Birmingham's Thomas McKeown, there were to be specialized general practitioners—GP paediatricians, GP mediatricians (caring for adults), GP geriatricians, and a GP psychiatrist (myself). Part of the time we would teach medical students, while for the remainder we provided a combination of general practice and specialist care for patients. As far as possible we were to look after the extended primary care needs of the local population and consume our own smoke. The whole initiative was supported by a dedicated mainframe computer capability to provide real-time clinical and population intelligence.

It was a stimulating time but there were problems reconciling the competing claims of the medical school and service as well as staffing issues.

Southampton was within spitting distance of the London School of Hygiene and Tropical Medicine and the local regional medical officer for Wessex, Sir John Revans, a man of great vision, was prepared to invest heavily in sending young clinicians to study public health at the school. It was time to make that step into public health and it was clear from the first week in the classroom in Gower Street in autumn 1976 that it was the right move.

The roots of public mental health

As public health in general has its roots in the Victorian age, so too does mental health, in which four phases can be identified. During the first phase in the eighteenth century the Elizabethan Poor Laws were administered through parish overseers to provide workhouses for the able-bodied poor, subject to the 'workhouse tests' which distinguished between the 'deserving' and the 'undeserving' poor. The parishes worked together in 'combinations' to provide care for the sick poor. The principle of 'lesser eligibility' was applied, whereby a condition of entering a workhouse was to have surrendered all your assets. These principles can still be found at work today, in particular with regard to the care of the frail elderly and those with dementia. The formation, dissolution, and reformation of Primary Care Trusts in recent years in England together with the creation of Clinical Commissioning Groups and their subsequent combination have clear resonances, as secular versions of a parish level of organization.

When it came to those labelled 'lunatics', people who we would now regard as suffering from severe and enduring mental illness, unable to care for themselves, there were a number of possible destinations:

1. The poorhouse, where 'pauper lunatics' were the responsibility of the parish overseer;

2. The local bridewell or house of correction for vagrants where no parish took responsibility;

3. Private madhouses run for profit by private proprietors who may well not be medically qualified;

4. Prisons where it was common for mentally ill people to be incarcerated alongside the mentally sane, then as now (insanity was first recognized as a defence against criminal charges in 1800); and

5. The Bethlehem Hospital in London, founded in 1247 by public subscription for pauper and non-pauper patients. According to Le Gassicke, 'its history was undistinguished from the humanitarian viewpoint and as late as 1770 anyone could pay to view the inmates as a form of public entertainment' (1).

In the second phase mass migration of paupers from rural areas to the growing cities began to overwhelm the poorhouses, and humanitarian interest in the care of the mentally ill was fuelled by public sympathy for King George III, who suffered from mental illness caused by porphyria, as well as by the sentiments of 'liberty, equality, and fraternity' which inspired the French Revolution from

1789. Scandals in private madhouses where patients were kept chained in rags and fed on gruel by proprietors who, having secured the year's funding, had no incentive to spend money on patient care, also played a part in demands for reform. The outcome was the County Asylum Act of 1808, which authorized the building of county asylums and which led to many being built over the next few decades. These took the form of whole communities complete with farms, workshops, and gymnasia and often accommodating thousands of patients. As rapidly as they opened they would fill up with patients who had often been kept hidden and out of sight by families unwilling to consign them to the brutal alternatives.

Over the next hundred years asylums themselves became less and less therapeutic and more seen as custodial institutions. It was against this background that a third phase, characterized by therapeutic optimism, can be identified after the Second World War. If the second phase had been influenced by the environmental and hygienist influences of the Victorian public health movement, this phase was possible because of the discoveries in pharmacological medicine. From the 1960s onwards the discovery of antidepressants and major tranquillizers revolutionized the management of patients suffering from major psychoses. Consequently, policy makers were influenced by projections on graphs that predicted the closure of all mental hospital beds within the foreseeable future and their replacement with community care. Unfortunately, this thinking failed to take into account different levels of severity of patients' impairment and was unduly influenced by the remarkable impact on some of the early patients treated with new medicines. It was also oversold inasmuch as the resources for proper community care were never forthcoming. Ensuing decades witnessed mental health services in increasing disarray, unable to deliver for children and adolescents, let alone for the 30 per cent of adults with mental health problems and the increasing numbers suffering with dementia and other organic brain conditions in an ageing society. Public health, wellbeing, and prevention which should characterize a fourth phase of mental public health barely had a look in. The characteristics of such a phase are only now emerging as the debate about mental ill-health being a leading cause of the burden of disease in populations gathers momentum.

It is difficult to make the case for the psychological theories and therapies that had followed the work of Sigmund Freud having made any impact at a population level until this period, having largely been confined to wealthy elites with functional neuroses and dealing with the problems of everyday life. Such whole population approaches to mental health as well as mental illness have been few and far between. However, it has become evident in recent years that cognitively based behavioural therapies may form part of an effective comprehensive approach to mental health that encompasses primary, secondary, and tertiary prevention (see Box 7.1).

Box 7.1 A glimpse into the recent past: St Nicholas Hospital, Gosforth, Northumberland

The Newcastle Borough Lunatic Asylum was opened in 1869 at Gosforth with accommodation for 159 patients and a full range of occupational facilities and activities.

When I worked there as a psychiatric registrar in the early 1970s it was on the cusp of change to community care, but still there were large dormitory 'back wards', each containing upwards of 30 patients. There were patients who had been hospitalized here for many years, even decades. As a registrar one of my duties was to administer electroconvulsive therapy (ECT) at the twice weekly ECT sessions. Long-term patients suffering from severe depression and other psychotic illnesses would regularly be brought down from their wards for so-called 'maintenance ECT'. They would have been receiving this treatment regularly for many years. My job was to hold the electrodes to their head and administer the treatment and record it in the treatment book.

St Nicholas Hospital was typical of so many of the county asylums in its splendid Victorian architecture. At the time I was working there the hospital management had arranged with the Laing Art Gallery in Newcastle to borrow large oil canvases which were displayed in the corridors. Within living memory, the physician superintendent had ridden round the grounds of the hospital in his coach and four (horses). The senior clinicians maintained the tradition of waiting on the patients with Christmas lunch; for the rest of the year the physician superintendents house was maintained by a ready supply of patient-servants.

Around the same time at the Learning Disabilities Hospital at Northgate in Northumberland I met a man in his 70s who had been put away as a teenager because his father was having trouble managing him. He was a benign and friendly person. I asked him if he would like to live outside in the community but after 60 years of institutional life the prospect terrified him. Some years later I led a review of health services on the Isle of Man. A survey of patients in Noble's Hospital in Douglas revealed one elderly woman who had been put away as a teenager for giving birth to a child outside marriage.

Towards public mental health

As a postgraduate student at the London School of Hygiene and Tropical Medicine validation for the move away from individual patient care came in the form of teaching from John Wing and Julian Leff from the Institute of Psychiatry, who taught social and transcultural psychiatry and anthropology at the school. This curriculum raised expectations about the prospects of an emphasis on the prevention agenda as it concerned mental health but such expectations were to be misplaced.

At that time students on the masters course had the enormous privilege of a two-year course, the second year being spent on a dissertation. The dissertation was a kind of blank cheque enabling you to pursue something of special interest that could be built on in future years. If you were wise, you chose something of interest to your sponsoring health authority and secure support for your chosen study. This was where my dilemma reasserted itself. What would be a suitable dissertation that majored on prevention and public mental health?

I took advice from as many people as I could find, including President of the Royal College of Psychiatrists, Sir Martin Roth. I drew a blank. The nearest anybody could get was the early diagnosis and treatment of major mental illness in the community. In public health terms this was secondary prevention, primary prevention being nowhere to be found.

Part of my student exposure in Newcastle had been to the paediatrician Christine Cooper and the family planning doctor Mary Peberdy, for whom the link between fertility control and family health and wellbeing was second nature. It was as a result of their influence that I was to add sexual health to my list of postgraduate qualifications. Mary Peberdy had introduced domiciliary family planning as a service for women who had already had many children but whose Roman Catholic husbands refused to allow them near the family planning clinic or to use contraception. Instead the consultations took place in the home while the husband was at work. Christine Cooper, for whom I worked as a junior, was equally certain about the benefits of family planning for women with large families and on one occasion when I was with her she interrupted her child health clinic to accompany a mother to the family planning clinic where she was fitted with an intrauterine contraceptive device on the spot. It was perhaps not such a surprise that I chose planned parenthood as my choice for a masters dissertation and I carried out a series of studies into family planning and abortion at the population level in Wessex Region of 3 million people.

In my subsequent career as an academic, as a regional and county director of public health, as World Health Organization adviser on Healthy Cities Project, and later as President of the UK's Faculty of Public Health, I have reconciled my angst in refocusing my psychiatric training upstream by considering that all public health work has ultimately to be judged by its impact on mental health and wellbeing running through it like a golden thread.

With both mental and physical health the default position often seems to be one of working backwards from a treatment focus towards one on prevention; the exception is when there is an emergency, disaster, or war when needs must apply a population-based triage model if harm is to be minimized. A key message from a 1980s short course for volunteers to humanitarian emergencies has stayed with me. If a small group of volunteers (perhaps doctors, nurses, and engineers) are drafted into a refugee camp, the first thing not to do is to spend all their time treating sick patients. Rather they are best advised to carry out a quick census of who is there and what skills you have, and to set about mobilizing the expertise and supporting it; asset-based community development, if you will. This is not the traditional medical model, based as it is on putting your nameplate up outside a consulting room and offering services to those who can afford to pay for them. There is no automatic concern for the denominator of those with unmet need or effort made to mobilizing existing assets for health as opposed to marketing your own services.

Take the example of child and adolescent psychiatry. Classic community surveys such as those on the Isle of Wight and in South London found that about 10 per cent of children and adolescents were suffering from such a level of emotional or conduct disorder as to require specialist help. In a borough of 500,000 population (perhaps 70,000 children and adolescents), this will equate to about 7,000 potential patients. In a fortunate district with a teaching hospital, about 1,000 of those could be adequately cared for by a typical child and adolescent mental health service. No district will have an adequate establishment of staff in the foreseeable future to meet current need. As a result grossly inequitable access to help is inevitable with those who are better connected being most likely to receive it and worse outcomes for the others who may also finish up in the criminal justice rather than the health care system. As Chinese leader Mao Tse Tung is reputed to have said, 'if the practice doesn't work the theory is wrong'. We are starting at the wrong end of the telescope and focusing on the wrong part of the pyramid of need. So what is an appropriate public health response?

In 1961 Gerald Caplan published a book titled *An Approach to Community Mental Health*. Caplan was educated at Manchester Medical School, the Tavistock Institute in London, and the Hadassah Centre in Jerusalem before moving to the USA. His work was hugely influential, not least with the programme of community mental health centres associated with President Kennedy. Caplan's book is as relevant and fresh today as when it was written, and it is a mystery to me why it has not provided a blueprint for mental health in the intervening years. Perhaps it is because it includes a (very sensible) chapter on 'ego' psychology, when British psychiatry has long been under the influence of biological theorists and psychopharmacology, important as they are.

What Caplan proposed was a comprehensive community approach to preventive psychiatry and the provision of services which builds on individual and community assets including those he calls 'care taking agents' together with those in special positions in everyday life. He included in this not only doctors, nurses, other clinical professionals, and social workers but also clergy, teachers, police officers, and others, advocating a system built on skilling up those in a position to play a protective and supportive role in everyday life as a front line.

Caplan identified administrative actions that can protect and support good mental health as well as personal and clinical interactions and redefined the role of those with specialist psychiatric expertise in building and supporting both capacity and capability for mental health and wellbeing. For myself, using the example of child and adolescent mental health, this translates into a life cycle approach that begins with planned parenthood, builds with support for parents that includes parenting classes, and ensures that all those in key interactions with parents and children have adequate skills to promote mental health and respond quickly to signs of distress. This extends to children themselves developing mental resilience and skills for mutual mental health assistance with their peers. The administrative component includes key action on wider determinants of mental health such as economic and social security, housing and access to good education, work and recreational opportunities.

If this is in place, the question arises as to what the formal health care system should be offering in both primary and specialist care and how best to meet the needs of patients with severe and enduring mental health problems requiring intensive or long-term intervention. Recent developments in improving access to psychological therapies (IAPTS) in the National Health Services point the way to a rational pathway of care that is rooted in the community.

One of the obstacles to adopting a comprehensive approach to mental health is the prevailing narrow and reductionist model of scientific evidence as illustrated by controversies over the concept of mental wellbeing as a researchable paradigm. For Caplan:

> Our lack of knowledge in regard to the significance of different factors has to be remedied by a continuation of existing research into aetiology. But, meanwhile preventive psychiatrists have been able to learn a lesson from public health colleagues in regard to handling of the problem of the multifactorial nature of the picture.... The incidence of cases of clinical tuberculosis, for example, in any community is no longer conceived of in public health circles as being merely dependent upon the single factor of the presence or absence of the tubercle bacillus. It is recognised that there are many complicated issues that will determine whether a particular person exposed to the germ will

contract the clinical disease: issues involving the virulence of the germ, host suscepti-bility, and various environmental factors. (2)

In public health we have learned to take a whole-systems approach to whole and subpopulations and to use multiple interventions acting across what Canadian Health Minister Lalonde called the 'health field'.

The list of factors of interest for protecting and improving mental health, mental wellbeing, and resilience, in addition to the proximal factors of personal security already mentioned and the managed challenges that enable people to grow and thrive, includes a set of constructs such as locus of control, self-esteem, and coherence. These can be difficult constructs to operationalize for research purposes, especially when they interact with complex systems, but tools can be developed; examples include the Rosenberg Self-Esteem Scale and those that measure sense of coherence. The concept of sense of coherence (SOC) was put forward by Aaron Antonovsky in 1979 to explain why some people become ill under stress whilst others remain healthy. It carries within it the three compo-nents of meaningfulness, manageability, and understandability and underpins the salutogenic approach which is at the heart of health promotion. Two scales have been developed to operationalize these concepts as valid research tools, a longer instrument and a shorter one, 'SOC13'. In recent years mixed methods such as those used in social return on investment have paved the way for prac-tical interventions based on pragmatic considerations (see Box 7.2).

Caplan's book concludes with a remarkably contemporary proposal for the development of comprehensive community psychiatry based on the ideas

Box 7.2 The Rosenberg Self-Esteem Scale (RSE)

1. On the whole I am satisfied with myself.
2. At times I think I am no good at all.
3. I think that I have a number of good qualities.
4. I am able to do things as well as most people.
5. I feel I do not have much to be proud of.
6. I certainly feel useless at times.
7. I feel that I am a person of worth, at least on an equal plane with others.
8. I wish I could have more respect for myself.
9. All in all, I am inclined to feel that I am a failure.
10. I take a positive attitude towards myself.

outlined above. I have come to the conclusion that in addition to those things which government can and should do to protect public mental health and lay the foundations for a thriving and resilient population, there are three approaches, tried and tested in recent years, that should be regarded as organizational forms and delivery systems:

1. 'Total place' and 'defined population' as developed through 'healthy cities, towns, and villages', 'healthy schools, workplaces', and other settings of everyday life.

2. Asset-based community development as proposed and expounded by John McKnight and his colleagues in Illinois. This approach maps and mobilizes the gifts and talents of individuals, families, and communities on the basis that:

   ◆ They are half-full, not half-empty.

   ◆ 'It takes a village to raise a child.'

   ◆ Ninety per cent of health and social care is lay care.

   Unless professional practice supports self-efficacy it can be part of the problem rather than part of the solution.

3. Community-orientated primary (and secondary) care, based on an epidemiological and sociological understanding of populations and responsibility for them.

I am optimistic that by adopting these approaches, grounded in a public health perspective, we can craft a system with a good chance of optimizing population mental health.

Organic mental illness, the coming challenge of dementia—a modern-day cholera?

We have seen earlier in this book how the threat of cholera epidemics in the nineteenth century galvanized communities into action through the organized efforts of society. The campaigning efforts of the Health of Towns Association resulted in a legal framework that empowered local authorities to act on the environmental conditions that predisposed to epidemics. Success in this work paved the way for an extension of local government into many areas of the provision services that improved the quality of life and health in urban areas. That story and the lessons it brings are highly relevant to the contemporary channels of dementia.

Dementia is now a global epidemic with an estimated 47 million sufferers worldwide rising to 75 million by 2030 and 135 million by 2050. Although we have become aware of the issue in developed countries in recent years, not least because of its association with an ageing population, a majority of dementia sufferers are to be found in the more populous low and middle income countries where access to social protection, support, and care are very limited. The term 'dementia' itself is used to describe a series of symptoms associated with biological decline caused by brain cell damage on thinking and memory skills which are sufficient to affect a person's everyday life. Cholera was an acute and potentially rapidly fatal disease and was typical of an era in which birth rates were high and longevity low. It was preventable by improving environmental conditions and ensuring that the population had access to safe water to drink. Although cholera is normally a water-borne disease, in 1847 Liverpool, such was the overcrowding in the slums, with as many as 16 people to a room, in small, airless back-to-back houses that it was spread from person to person.

Dementia, on the other hand, is representative of the modern pattern of disease in the twenty-first century in which we have low birth rates, increasing longevity, but also accumulations of long-term conditions which are sometimes or often preventable. The paradox of these modern conditions is that the more we are able to provide palliation, which increases survival, the greater becomes their prevalence and the impact of the burden of care to society. When I was a medical student in the 1960s the average life of a person diagnosed with dementia was 3–5 years; today it could be more like 10. Consider the potential impact on health and social services of many thousands of people surviving with dementia for an extra 5 years. As with any health problem, when viewed through a public health prism, the challenge is to optimize the balance between prevention, treatment, and care. With dementia we seem at the moment to be narrowly focused on the possibilities and prospects for early diagnosis and treatment to the detriment of optimizing both prevention and mitigation. If we are to rebalance this, we must take a whole-systems approach, not just to prevention, treatment, and care but to the biological, the social, and the environmental. This is where place-based approaches such as the WHO Healthy Cities initiative comes in with its integrative focus on creating urban habitats to support health and wellbeing. Local government with its responsibilities for the environment, housing, community development, and cultural activities is at the heart of this mission.

Without wishing to ignore the possibility that treatment options may emerge for the different types of dementia and being aware that preparations as varying as statins, aspirin, and viagra (reaching the parts that other medicines don't reach) are claimed to impact on the condition, in practical terms and in the current state of knowledge it is prudent to increase the emphasis on prevention and mitigation. We should do this if for no other reason than that to spend too much effort on treatment without optimizing prevention could lead to an accumulation of avoidable morbidity and a crippling impact on health and social care. In 2007 Cumbria, with a population of 500,000, there were around 7,000 people identified as living with dementia, with a projected doubling over the following 10–15 years, in part because of the numbers of elderly people retiring into the county. With a population profile that included only two young people entering the labour market for every three retiring, the difficulties in providing enough carers into the future loomed large.

Population ageing is the main driver of the projected increases around the world with the numbers expected to increase across Europe by slightly less than twofold between 2015 and 2050. The incidence increases exponentially with increasing age, doubling with every six years increase in age from 3.1 per 1000 at age 60–4 to 175 per 1000 at age 95 plus. All current projections of the scale of this epidemic assume that the age- and gender-specific prevalence will not vary over time and that the increases in the numbers of older people will be what drives the projected increases. However, as already indicated, changes in either incidence rate or the survival of patients could impact on the changing prevalence. A decline in age-specific incidence in the majority of patients where there is no or little genetic component is possible with changes in the known lifestyle and cardiovascular risk factors. Alzheimer's disease, where there may be a genetic component, is the most common type of the disease, with vascular dementia usually involving diabetes or hypertension making up much of the rest. The strongest evidence for causal associations with dementia are those of low education in early life, high blood pressure in middle age, and alcohol, smoking, and diabetes across the life course. Modelling work suggests that a 20 per cent reduction in risk factors could lead to a 15 per cent reduction in the prevalence of dementia. Such a reduction could be achieved by vigorous population-based health promotion programmes.

From the management and mitigation point of view there is an increasing body of knowledge about dementia-friendly environments including those in clinics, hospitals, and care homes. However, it is changes in town planning, in neighbourhood design, and in the environments of people's own homes that can make the most difference in lengthening the period of independent living together with the 'organized efforts of society' in the form of family, friends, neighbours, and volunteers supported by the statutory services. Experience from Scandinavia shows that this is possible through the provision of sheltered housing at the heart of communities where people have spent their lives. These are often to be found in proximity to neighbourhood health centres from which nurses and social workers can readily provide light touch supervision and oversight for folk whose skills for everyday living are on a downward path.

Extra care for those with advanced dementia is often located nearby, making it possible to maintain intergenerational contact, including through projects involving local schoolchildren.

Imagine the projected 10,000 dementia sufferers in a county like Cumbria being able to live in their own homes for an extra 1–2 years if the organized efforts of society, led and facilitated by the local authority in real partnership with citizens, were to line up all the ducks in a row:

◆ Dementia-friendly homes and neighbourhoods;

◆ A big society of an asset-based community development kind involving the support of family members, neighbours, and volunteers; and

◆ A strengthened capacity of community and social care.

There would be a need for 10–20,000 less patient-years of hospital, residential, or care home beds. Think of what that means in terms not only of professional staff and costs but also the quality of life of sufferers and their loved ones.

From the dancing manias of the Middle Ages to epidemic suicide: contagion and public health

A paradox of clinical psychiatry has been its failure to give much consideration to social psychological phenomena and to contagion. I can find little mention of contagion or of epidemics in the 904 pages of my old standard textbook of *Clinical Psychiatry* by Eliot Slater and Martin Roth dating from the early 1970s, yet history is rich with examples. Perhaps the most dramatic and well known are the examples of the so-called 'dancing mania' of the Middle Ages as described in the classic account by Hecker. This was a social phenomenon that occurred in Europe between the fourteenth and seventeenth centuries involving sometimes thousands of people dancing erratically for long periods and spreading across large areas, especially in France and the Netherlands, before eventually subsiding. Various names were given to the phenomenon including St. John's and St Vitus' dance and it was attributed among other things to spider bites, ergot poisoning from rye bread, and hysteria. It seems to have occurred especially under conditions of economic and social hardship including times of famine and during the plague and sometimes involved groups of religious pilgrims. Hecker includes accounts of episodes that occurred after the Black Death, when people danced, screamed, foamed at the mouth, and leaped in the air doing the St Vitus' dance. During this period there was also the Flagellant movement in which people publicly scourged themselves in European cities. According to some commentators it was made worse by attempts to shake it off by the use of musicians to accompany the dancing; this may have contributed to the origins of the story of the Pied Piper of Hamelin. Novelist Isaac Bashevis Singer draws on the stories, together with those relating to millennial movements, to describe false prophets with ulterior motives who exploit the naivety of peasants during such periods.

In the eighteenth century an epidemic in which nuns mewed in unison for several hours at a time occurred in a French convent. This ended only when they were threatened with being whipped. There was also a biting mania on the continent at this time and an epidemic of hysterical behaviour in a Lancashire cotton mill in Hodden Bridge. Mill girls were in convulsions for hours on end and had to be prevented from tearing their hair and hitting their heads on the walls and floor.

Norman Cohn, in his history of popular religious and social movements in Europe of the Middle Ages, paints a vivid picture of mass phenomena which were prompted by biblical beliefs focused on the end of the world, as predicted in the Old Testament of the Bible. Incidents such as these are familiar to us in relation to recent disastrous outcomes involving charismatic leaders such as James Jones in Georgetown, Guyana and the siege in Waco, Texas in 1993, in which many people died.

In recent times many reports of epidemics of hysterical reactions have appeared in the medical literature from around the world involving a wide range of symptoms. Often these have occurred in institutional settings where there appear to have been high levels of stress. Symptoms include weakness, sweating, trembling, crying, itching, headaches, sore throat or eyes, nausea, pain in the abdomen or limbs, over-breathing leading to muscle spasms, trance-like states, fainting, and collapsing. In some cultures screaming and laughing have been reported. In the Far East epidemics of the culture-bound syndrome 'Koro' have been reported in which the subject believes that his penis will disappear into his abdomen with fatal consequences. In 1945, the midwestern community in Mattoon, Illinois, came to believe that a phantom anaesthetist was prowling the town and raping women. Vigilante patrols were set up until it transpired that it had just been a rumour.

Public health workers are much more likely to find themselves dealing with lower levels of psychological contagion but this can extend to clusters of people taking their own lives. My own interest was prompted by a seemingly benign incident involving a juvenile jazz band on 13 July 1980 at a contest in a field in Mansfield, South Yorkshire. Two-hundred and eighty children collapsed in rapid succession and were taken to hospital. A striking feature was the speed of the episode, with children catching their friends as they fell. Symptoms included shaking, nausea, vomiting, running eyes, sore throat, and a metallic taste in the mouth. Environmental investigations focused on food poisoning and an ice-cream salesman was mobbed by angry parents but in the end the children recovered quickly and no cause was found. It was concluded that the combination of overdressed children on a hot day in a competitive environment had led to a domino effect.

Often outbreaks of this kind are explosive in onset but last for only a few days. The beliefs and reactions of the principal participants in an outbreak are important in understanding its nature; account must be taken of the victims, the observers, and the mass media. The development of illness among the initial 'index' cases under conditions of stress in a pre-disposed population leads to the rapid development of rumour, and the rapid expectation that something is going to happen. The ensuing anxiety can give rise to vague symptoms and the perception and labelling of the symptoms may be influenced by the prevailing mood. They can easily be seen as manifestations of illness.

Sometimes epidemics of apparent hysteria can follow outbreaks of serious physical illness as happened in Blackburn in 1965. An outbreak of over-breathing with pins and needles and muscle spasms followed an epidemic of polio in the town. The most controversial outbreak of this kind was probably that which occurred at the Royal Free Hospital in London in 1955 and led to the hospital being closed. At the time it was attributed to an unknown infectious disease but when the data were subsequently re-examined, it was concluded that epidemic hysteria was a much more likely explanation. This view was very unpopular with medical and nursing commentators. A special meeting was held at the Royal Society of Medicine with an audience that seems to have been lacking in psychiatrists, a vote was taken, and it was concluded that there was insufficient evidence to support the psychological view (see Box 7.3).

Suicide: its epidemic manifestations and its prevention

Around 6,000 people take their own lives each year in the United Kingdom; around three times as many as are killed on the nation's roads. Male rates, at around 19 per hundred thousand, are almost four times female rates but female rates have been increasing in recent years. The highest rates in men are under the age of 44 and in women in the older age of 45–74.

Suicide may be at once an act of self-directed violence, destroying the individual and simultaneously an act of aggression against others. Its patterns vary at different times, as do the methods used, but ready access to methods is one important pointer to possible prevention efforts. Accounting for several thousand deaths annually in England and Wales, consummated suicide is correlated with male sex, increasing age, widowhood, single and divorced state, childlessness, high density of population, residence in large towns, a high standard of

---

Box 7.3 An outbreak of vague symptoms in a girls' school

In the spring of 1979, 45 of 103 residential pupils in an English girls' school developed symptoms of headache, sore throat, abdominal pain, tiredness, weakness, pallor, and tearfulness.

The girls completed a symptom questionnaire and were physically examined. A table was produced for those with symptoms and with physical signs.

Symptoms and signs were compared with pathological findings, attendance rates at the school sick bay, and neuroticism scores. Patients ($n = 45$) were compared with the other girls ($n = 57$).

The patients were more frequent attenders at the sick bay. Except at age 14, the patients who had no positive findings had a higher neuroticism score than the other girls; the younger patients had higher neuroticism scores than non-patients. Some of the girls had common infectious diseases but not constituting one clinical entity. The patients had on average 8.1 symptoms compared with 1.5 in the other girls.

After the school holidays only one girl was still unwell. She had been the first case in the outbreak and the other girls were 'like her'. Early in the new term she was diagnosed as having haematocolpos (intact hymen with retained blood), giving rise to a temperature which returned to normal with appropriate treatment.

It was felt that use of the word 'hysterical' was not helpful to describe the patients in the outbreak, and a diagnosis of benign myalgic encephalomyelitis was made.

---

living, economic crisis, alcohol and drug consumption, history of broken home in childhood, mental disorder, and physical illness. Although men are historically more likely to resort to violent methods to take their own lives there is some indication of a convergence of male and female behaviours in recent years.

The earliest work on the epidemiology of suicide was the remarkably sophisticated study by the French sociologist Durkheim which led him to the belief that suicide could only be understood in the context of the society in which the individual was living. Durkheim felt that suicide was inevitable in any society but that it would be more likely to occur when the social structure and the social norms led to the failure of the group to support the individual—the so-called anomic suicide. The anthropologist Margaret Meade described a specific example of this from the South Pacific where suicidal individuals would take to sea in a small boat without oars to bring them back; they were dependent on the expressed solidarity of their community in retrieving them.

Durkheim also described egotistical suicide as being when the individual had no concern for the group and altruistic suicide such as that of Captain Oates of the Antarctic, when it is a sacrifice to maintain the continuity of the group.

From the clinical point of view extreme personality types are more likely to take their own lives, especially if they suffer from psychotic depression or other serious and enduring mental condition. Patients in profound states of depression may feel overwhelming guilt driving them to self-destruction whilst those with schizophrenic illness may carry out their action in response to their auditory hallucinations. The combination of personality disorder with alcohol and drugs produces particular risk and there are times of life such as adolescence when mood swings are common and later life when the attrition of constant loss can impact on the will to live. A high proportion of patients with depression who take their lives have seen a doctor or other clinical professional in the days before suicide. The prevention of suicide at a population level is an important part of the public health task (see Box 7.4).

The role of the media in epidemic suicide

The role of the media in propagating epidemics and clusters of suicides has already been touched on. One of the most notorious recent examples of this was the spate of deaths that occurred in Bridgend in South Wales, involving young people, and starting in January 2007. By December 2008 there had been 26 suicides, all but one by hanging. Although the police found no evidence to link the deaths, the parents of the young people concerned accused the media of 'glamorizing ways of taking one's life to young people'.

Research into this issue has shown that sensational reporting of the deaths of younger men by violent methods is more likely to be followed by similar events in time and geography. The recommendations for responsible reporting are that it should be low key without sensationalizing or glamorizing and not describe the method or location. Following my own experience of researching the increase in suicide deaths by immolation I campaigned with local media, wherever I was working and with various degrees of success, to try and persuade editors to adopt responsible best practice. On one occasion in Cheshire the local paper actually carried a photograph on its front page of where a young person had hanged themselves; fortunately, there were no copycat events on that occasion. On the other hand the then editor of the *Manchester Evening News*, Paul Horrocks, with whom I enjoyed a good relationship and who was well aware of my concerns, took the opportunity of hosting the Press Complaints

Box 7.4 Suicide by fire: An example of an epidemic

On 2 October 1978, Lynette Phillips, a 24-year-old Australian heiress, burned herself to death in front of the Palais de Nations in Geneva. Lynette was a member of a religious sect called PROUT (Progressive Utilization Theory) and a follower of the sect's charismatic leader, P. R. Sarkar.

Within days it became apparent that other people, only a few of whom were sect members, were taking similar action. Over the 12-month period from 2 October 1978 to 1 October 1979, 82 people in England and Wales took their lives by this method. This compared with an average of 23 each year between 1963 and 1978.

There were no suicides committed as political gestures and the picture was one of people who were known to be mentally disturbed. Ninety per cent had ongoing psychiatric problems of whom half had spent time as a psychiatric inpatient. Previous suicide attempts had often been made. However, at least one-third of the victims appeared to be responding to an immediate problem social situation such as family break-up.

For many of the victims, death was not instantaneous, only 31% dying immediately and 29% surviving over 24 hours, with some living several weeks before succumbing from shock, burns, bronchopneumonia, or renal failure.

There can be little doubt that the spread of this specific epidemic must have been mediated by news coverage with deaths being widely reported, often in graphic detail.

Commission meeting in Manchester to invite me to address them. The outcome of this was a willingness to accept a tighter code of practice (see Box 7.5).

Preventing suicide, the example of Cumbria

In my director of public health report for Cumbria for 2008, I recorded differences in rates between the six districts of the county and suggested that there was scope for reducing the annual toll. One unusual characteristic was the number of people who travelled from around the country to take their lives in beautiful environment of the Lake District, perhaps because it held some special significance for them. A priority coming out of that report was to develop a suicide prevention strategy which would mobilize best practise to make a difference. This work was led from the public health team by Jane Mathieson

Box 7.5 What's the story? Reporting mental health and suicide. A resource for journalists and editors. (http://www.shift.org.uk/mediahandbook).

The do's and don'ts of covering suicide

- Seek help from … organizations for expert advice, information … or individuals who have direct knowledge of suicide.

- Take care to avoid giving excessive details about the method of suicide used because it may result in copycat suicide.

- Always include details of an appropriate helpline, such as Samaritans.

- Suicide was decriminalized in (the UK), in 1961, so it is inaccurate to use the term 'commit suicide'. Use alternatives such as 'took his own life', 'die by suicide', or 'complete suicide'.

- Suicide is complex. People decide to take their own lives for many different reasons. It is misleading to suggest a simplistic cause-and-effect explanation.

- Avoid sensational headlines or language that glorify or romanticize the act of suicide.

- Don't use dramatic photographs, footage, or images related to a suicide.

and Elaine Church in partnership with the Cumbria Partnership Trust which provided mental health services.

In January 2009 a wide range of agencies, together with service users and carers, were brought together to form the Cumbria Suicide Prevention Reference Group. Almost two years later a detailed strategy was produced which started from the recognition that with approximately 50 suicides each year, the county was experiencing 10–15 more events than might be expected from the national average, and that a proportion of these could be prevented by concerted action. The context for the work was the Department of Health national strategy 'Preventing Suicide in England', which identified six key areas for action.

1. Reduce the risk of suicide in high-risk groups.
2. Tailor approaches to improve mental health in specific groups.
3. Reduce access to means of suicide.

4. Provide better information and support to those bereaved or affected by suicide.

5. Support the media in delivering sensitive approaches to suicide and suicidal behaviour.

6. Support research, data collection, and monitoring.

The outcome was a comprehensive work programme which segmented the range, type, and location of consummated suicides in the county and pursued specific initiatives to reduce them in the future. Examples included:

1. MIND, a mental health charity, delivered extensive suicide training on suicide awareness to staff across a number of sectors.

2. Samaritans and Network Rail worked together to target high-risk areas and environments with environmental measures. This included signage in suicide hotspots with Samaritan contact numbers, an evidence-based measure, and construction to prevent jumping.

3. The public health team, together with other agencies, funded the establishment of a self-help group 'Survivors of Bereavment by Suicide' (SOBS) (see Box 7.6).

End of life issues, a public health approach

As the population ages, together with the major social changes that have occurred in recent decades, with changes in the nature of the nuclear family and our way of life, concern has focused on the medical, social, psychological, and environmental issues relating to the quality of our final days and weeks. 'Dignity and Comfort at the Time of Death' was identified in 'Health in Mersey' as a priority back in 1984. What we know is that most people who are nearing the end of their lives would like to die at home whilst their intimates tend to be much less certain how to respond and what the options are. As a consequence a high proportion of people are still dying in clinical institutional settings where the experience of all concerned may be very variable.

Public awareness of the issues involved has increasingly been identified as a priority worldwide. In England an End of Life Care strategy identified a need to raise the profile of end of life care and a national coalition, Dying Matters, has worked to encourage community education initiatives.

In Cumbria, using an approach developed in California by Mary Mathieson, a systematic programme of 'Conversations for Life' was commissioned around the county over a two-year period. Co-branded with the National Health Service and funded from the public health budget the project aimed to improve

Box 7.6 The death of Helena Farrell

On 4 January 2013, a Friday evening a 15-year-old young woman from Kendal, Helena Farrell, took her own life in a beauty spot frequented by local teenagers. A popular pupil and talented musician she had gone to pains to create an environment of great poignancy. Within a couple of hours word of Helena's death was widespread on social media; friends created a montage of photos set to music on YouTube, which received over 70,000 views, and Facebook tribute pages were created.

This incident prompted fears of creating an environment in which copycat behaviour could be initiated and the decision was taken by the Public Health Team to call a Health Gold Unusual Incident Meeting. This was not well received by the County Social Services Department for reasons which remained obscure.

A comprehensive set of measures was put in place including the following:

1. Meetings and telephone discussions were held with the editors and controllers of the local print and live media explaining the importance of restrained reporting and the need to keep within published reporting guidelines.

2. A 24-hour telephone advice line with counselling support was set up and run by the local mental health service provider acting in conjunction with the Samaritans.

3. Support was provided directly to the staff of the school at which Helena had been a student and to other local schools, and indirect support was provided to the students of those schools through staff training carried out by the Samaritans.

4. Family doctors and other community health workers were briefed on the situation and encouraged to be alert to signs of distress in family, intimates, and professionals.

5. An accelerated pathway of referral was established for anybody showing signs of exceptional distress. This had some uptake.

6. A system of enhanced surveillance of contacts with services among those possibly affected was established. This enabled the impact of this distressing incident to be monitored.

7. There were no consequential suicides among young people in the area in the ensuing weeks.

awareness and encourage conversations about people's end of life wishes. The objectives were to:

- Break the taboo of talking about death and dying while healthy;
- Help the public consider options and improve access to local resources; and
- Support people to learn how to begin conversations to influence their care in the future when their time came; there was an emphasis on 'breaking the silence'.

This programme was very well received by a wide variety of groups, both professional and lay, and began a process which continues and has become part of a much wider international initiative drawing on an asset-based philosophy and place-based initiates.

Better mental health for all

In recent years the recognition of the importance of mental health as a public health issue has finally begun to create a momentum for change. In the United Kingdom much of this has been led by the Mental Health Foundation with a significant part being played by *The Times* newspaper, which has run a campaign for mental health to be taken seriously over a number of years.

In 2016, in my final year as president of the UK Faculty of Public Health, I decided to adopt 'Better Mental Health for All' as a theme for the year, returning to my roots in mental health 40 years before, in a wish to contribute to this new dynamic. One outcome of this work was a commissioned report which was published by the Faculty of Public Health and the Mental Health Foundation, led by Sarah Stewart-Brown, a long-time champion of public mental health.

The report, 'Better Mental Health', brought together many of the themes which I have identified in this chapter, using the organizing principle of the human lifecycle situated within the settings of everyday life. Beginning with the epidemiology of what we know about mental health and illness the case was made for a strategic and systematic approach to the promotion and protection of public mental health and painted a picture of what will prove to be some of the first steps on a most important journey.

References

1. **Le Gassicke, John.** The early history of the asylums of Newcastle upon Tyne. *Newcastle Medical Journal* **31**(1) (1969), 36–41.
2. **Caplan, Gerald.** *An Approach to Community Mental Health.* London: Tavistock, 1961.

Further Reading

Antonovsky, A. *Unravelling the Mystery of Health: How People Manage Stress and Stay Well.* San Francisco: Jossey-Bass, 1987.

Ashton, John R. *Everyday Psychiatry.* Update Books, 1980.

Ashton, John R. The challenges of positive mental health. Journal of the Royal Society for the Promotion of Health **124**(3) (2004), 108–9.

Ashton, John R. Plans, hopes and ideas for mental health. *B J Psych Bulletin* **40** (2016), 1–4.

Ashton, John R. Two cheers for May's discovery of child and adolescent mental health. BMJ **356**: j335.

Ashton, John R., and **Stuart Donnan**. Suicide by burning as an epidemic phenomenon: an analysis of 82 deaths and inquests in England and Wales in 1978-9. Psychological Medicine **11** (1981),735–9.

Berridge, Virginia. *Demons: Our changing attitudes to alcohol, tobacco and drugs.* Oxford: Oxford University Press, 2013.

Brown, Jean S., **Alyson M. Learmonth**, and **Catherine J. Mackereth**. *Promoting Public Mental Health and Well-Being.* London: Jessica Kingsley, 2015.

Caplan, Gerald. *An Approach to Community Mental Health.* London: Tavistock, 1961.

Caplan, Gerald. *Population Oriented Psychiatry.* New York: Human Sciences Press, 1989.

Cohen, Stanley. *Folk Devils and Moral Panics.* Paladin, 1973.

Cohn, Norman. *The Pursuit of the Millenium.* London: Secker and Warburg, 1957.

Cooper, David. *Psychiatry and Anti-Psychiatry.* Paladin, 1970.

Cumbria Partnership NHS Foundation Trust. *Suicide Prevention Plan.* Cumbria Partnership NHS Foundation Trust, 2013.

Department of Health Mental Health Division. *New Horizons: A Shared Vision for Mental Health.* London: HM Government, 2009.

Durkheim, Emile. *Suicide. A Study in Sociology.* London: Routledge and Kegan Paul, 1975.

Gladwell, Malcolm. *The Tipping Point. How little Things Can make a Big Difference.* Boston: Little, Brown, 2002.

Health in Cumbria. The Annual Report of the Director of Public Health. Cumbria County Council and Cumbria Primary Care Trust, 2008.

Hecker, J. F. C. *The Dancing Mania of the Middle Ages.* New York: Burt Franklin, 1970.

Knifton, Lee, and **Neil Quinn** (eds). *Public Mental Health.* London: McGraw Hill, Open University Press, 2013.

Le Gassicke, John. The early history of the asylums of Newcastle upon Tyne. *Newcastle Medical Journal* **31**(1) (1969), 36–41.

Lukes, Steven. *Emile Durkheim: His Life and Work: A Historical and Critical Study.* London: Penguin Books, 1975.

Marching bands and mass hysteria: A psychological look at the 'Mansfield Sunday' syndrome. New Society (1980), 166–7.

Matthiesen, Mary E. *Dying to Make a Difference.* CreateSpace, 2016.

Mathieson, Mary, **Katherine Froggatt**, **Elaine Owen**, and **John R. Ashton**. End of life conversations and care: an asset-based model for community engagement. BMJ Supportive and Palliative Care **0** (2014), 1–7.

May, Peter G. R., Stuart P. B. Donna, John R. Ashton, Marie M. Ogilvie, and Christopher J. Rolles. Personality and perception in benign myalgic encephalomyelitis. *The Lancet* 316(8204) (1980), 1122–4.

Mental Health Foundation. *A New Way Forward. A World with Good Mental Health For All.* London: Mental Health Foundation, 2016.

Mental Health Foundation. *Better Mental health For All. A Public Health Approach to Mental Health Improvement.* London: Faculty of Public Health, and Mental Health Foundation, 2016.

Morris, Pauline. *Put Away.* International Library of Sociology. London: Routledge, 1998.

Osorno, Jairo, Leif Svanstrom, and Jan Beskow. *Community Suicide Prevention.* Stockholm: Karolinska Institut, 2010.

Slater, Eliot, and Martin Roth. *Clinical Psychiatry.* London: Bailliere, Tindall and Cassell, 1970.

Szasz, Thomas S. *The Myth of Mental Illness.* Paladin, 1972.

Taylor, Lord, and Sidney Chave. *Mental Health and Environment.* London: Longmans, 1964.

What's the Story: Reporting Mental Health and Suicide. A Resource for Journalists and Editors. Available at http://www.mediawise.org.uk/wp-content/uploads/2011/03/Whats-the-story-reporting-mental-health-and-suicide.pdf.

Chapter 8

Healthy cities

Success has 100 parents; failure is an orphan

When a small group of us sat around a Copenhagen table on a snowy January day in 1986, we had no way of knowing that the proposed World Health Organization 'Healthy Cities' Project would acquire such momentum. Over 30 years later it is still going strong, has spread around the world involving thousands of cities, towns, and villages, and has become a real force in shaping of urban life and health in the twenty-first century.

Many streams of consciousness and endeavour flowed together to create the impulse for the project but the idea dates from a Toronto conference, 'Beyond Health Care', in 1984. This was a review of the Lalonde Report, which had argued for a new approach to public health. The idea of focusing on the city as a context was picked up by Ilona Kickbusch, head of the Health Promotion Unit at WHO, and on her return to Copenhagen she planted a potent seed. Whilst passing through Copenhagen in the summer of 1985, I called in on Ilona, who had heard of our work in Liverpool, and she asked me to coordinate the first stages of the project. It was a life-changing moment for me and the beginning of an extraordinary journey.

Following the Alma Ata Declaration on Primary Health Care, initial progress in creating a new momentum for public health had been slow despite the adoption of the Health for All Strategy by WHO member states in 1981. For many countries the initiative appeared to stop there. It seemed to be a common view that WHO existed as a vehicle for the developed world to offer advice to others and that there were few implications for policy and practice at home. The untoward consequences of this were all too often the exporting of hospital-heavy health care systems, although the Alma Ata concept of the 'core functions' of primary health care was beginning to offer a more sustainable vision for resource-poor countries. On the other hand, Europe could not identify an equivalent successful initiative to the recent global eradication of smallpox and some in Copenhagen were keen to find an equally potent flagship intervention. With increasing resource constraints and rapid and global urbanization appearing on the radar, Ilona was quick to see the potential of a public health initiative focusing on the continent's cities.

During the winter of 1985/6 the WHO European Office developed the initial concept of a limited project involving four to six cities to pilot whole-system, city-wide approaches to 'the New Public Health' and I was invited to facilitate it. This would involve local action plans based on Health For All principles. The work of Trevor Hancock and his colleagues in Toronto, together with our own work in Liverpool, was seen as providing tangible examples of the way forward. In addition the 1984 Toronto conference had its origins in a growing awareness of the need for 'healthy public policies' to counteract the tendency towards victim-blaming lifestyle approaches; these had become commonplace in many countries in contrast to the systematic, policy-oriented, and whole-population initiatives being pioneered in Scandinavia, especially Finland. One Toronto paper, 'The Healthy City', provided a specific focus for the new synthesis which might 'bring together an ecological and holistic approach to health together with the WHO "Health For All" Strategy'.

Many people have invested significant energy in taking forward the healthy city idea since it was first mooted, one of the strengths of the project since the outset being its embrace of a multidisciplinary approach. Sitting around that Copenhagen table on January 13th the perspectives represented included town planning and architecture, environmental health, social and political science, primary health care and public health, health services management, mental health, and journalism. Father of the group, psychiatrist, and urban planner from the University of California–Berkeley Len Duhl represented a link with President John Kennedy's 'Model Towns' initiative in 1960s America, where Duhl had been a presidential adviser. At one point in the meeting Len drew attention to the fact that each of us had at some point changed disciplines, arguing that the ability to approach urban health from multiple perspectives would be a prerequisite for success (see Box 8.1).On my return to England, London School of Hygiene Professor Jerry Morris drew my attention to the achievements of the UK Health of Towns Association of the 1840s, pointing out that we were proposing a contemporary equivalent.

This group was soon to be joined by Dutch ecological town planner Tjeerd Deelstra, environmental health experts Eric Giroult and Michael Suess from WHO and Bob Tanner from the UK, policy analyst Ron Draper from Canada, German public health academic Gunter Conrad, Danish architect and planner Marie Bistrup, and UK journalist Jill Turner. Later still the cast list broadened as Marilyn Rice led the role out in the Americas from the Pan American Health Organization in Washington; Chris Gates, Ashley Files, Jo Haley, Joan Twist, Beverly Flynn, Melinda Rider, and John Parr took responsibility in the United States; and Fran Baum, Antoinette Ackerman, Judy White, Richard Hicks, Hero Weston, Val Brown, Lewis Kaplan, Louise Croot, and Janet Takarangi in

Box 8.1 The Healthy Cities Planning Group, 13–17 January 1986

John Ashton, public health physician, psychiatrist, and family doctor
Keith Barnard, health services manager
Ian Burton, UNESCO
Len Duhl, psychiatrist and town planner
Trevor Hancock, public health physician, urbanist, and futurologist
Constantino Sakellarides, public health physician and specialist in
    elderly care
Ilona Kickbusch, political and social scientist
Harry Vertio, primary care physician

Australia and New Zealand. In the Eastern Mediterranean Office of WHO in Alexandria, Dr M. I. Sheikh and Q. Khosh Chasm adapted the project for the Middle East and for Iran whilst the enthusiastic promotion of Healthy Cities by former Medical Officer of Health S. H. Lee would lead in time to complete coverage of Hong Kong by healthy city projects and penetration far into mainland China and across the Western Pacific region. At the WHO Head Office in Geneva Greg Goldstein together with Drs Tarimo and Tabibzadeh were quick to see the value of Healthy Cities in the rapidly urbanizing cities of the Indian subcontinent and Africa where local conferences and initiatives followed. By 1991 British Chief Medical Officer Sir Donald Acheson was sufficiently taken by Healthy Cities that as chairman of the World Health Assembly Technical Discussions he chose as a theme for the discussions that of 'Health For All in the Face of Rapid Urban Development'. I was flattered to be asked by Sir Donald to act as his rapporteur for the meeting.

The context for 'Healthy Cities'

The rationale for focusing on public health in urban areas was strong. By the 1980s there was a dawning realization that within 20 years 75 per cent of Europeans and the majority of the world's population would be living in large towns or cities and that smaller communities were also facing demographic and other environmental and spatial challenges. Some Third World cities such as Mexico City, Sao Paula, Rio de Janeiro, Bombay, Calcutta, Jakarta, Seoul, Cairo, and Manila were already reaching extremely large sizes with populations of 15–20 million becoming not uncommon. The problems of British cities 150 years previously were now being found in these cities, albeit on a much larger scale and with much greater consequences. However, some things were very different especially with the advent of technologies such as antibiotics, immunization, and other medical measures which held the prospect of short-circuiting the trajectories which had been followed so many years before in Europe. In addition many of these twentieth-century conurbations already had, for better or worse, elaborate public sector organizations that might be deployed to ameliorate the growing pressures.

At this time too, people were beginning to make the connection between the urban condition and the growing eco-crisis confronting the planet. According to the chairperson of the World Commission on the Environment, former Norwegian Prime Minister and Director General of the World Health Organization Gro Harlem Brundtland:

> There are also environmental trends that threaten to radically alter the planet, that threaten the lives of many species upon it, including the human species. Each year another 6 million hectares of productive dry land turns into worthless desert. Over three decades, this would amount to an area roughly as large as Saudi Arabia. More than 11 million hectares of forests are destroyed yearly, and this, over three decades would equal an area the size of India. Much of the forest is converted to low-grade farmland unable to support the farmers who settle it. In Europe, acid precipitation kills forests and lakes and damages the artistic and architectural heritage of nations; it may have acidified vast tracts of soil beyond reasonable hope of repair. The burning of fossil fuels puts into the atmosphere carbon dioxide, which is causing gradual global warming. This 'greenhouse effect' may by early next century have increased average global temperatures enough to shift agricultural production areas, raise sea levels, to flood coastal cities, and disrupt national economies. Other industrial gases threaten to deplete the planet's protective ozone shield to such an extent that the number of human and animal cancers would rise sharply and the oceans' food chain would be disrupted. Industry and agriculture put toxic substances into the human food chain and into underground water tables beyond reach of cleansing.' (1)

There was at this time an increasing, but by no means uncontested, realization of the need to grapple with these self-induced crises which were beginning to threaten global ecosystems. These crises were largely the results of major lifestyle changes and the actions of politicians and city dwellers impacting on patterns of agriculture and world development. It was becoming apparent that the mechanistic, engineering solutions to the sanitary problems of cities could not be adequately dealt with using Victorian approaches. In that sense the 'sanitary idea', so important in the past had been found wanting. Moving sewage and solid waste away from its origin and dumping it elsewhere may have bought time when a few, relatively small European cities were involved. However, when a greater proportion of a much bigger population was implicated, it was a recipe for ecological catastrophe as the carrying capacity of biological systems became overloaded. The shift from sanitary to ecological thinking had significant implications for the way life was lived in cities and for the underpinning policies. The 'ecological idea', of understanding how complex natural systems interact, and of working with them, rather than attempting to subjugate them, carries with it at least as powerful a motivational potential as the 'sanitary idea' had in the 1840s. The challenge continues to be to move towards cities and towns which are based on sound ecological principles and which can respond to changing demographics, expectations, and realities.

Beginnings: the Lisbon Healthy Cities Conference, 7–10 April 1986

The first formal activity of the Healthy Cities Project was marked by a conference in Lisbon just three months after that January meeting in Copenhagen. The opportunity that presented itself was an existing event that had been planned to showcase current work led by the Lisbon City Council, supported by Constantino Sakellarides from the National School of Public Health. Delegates and advisers from over 20 cities gathered in one of Europe's most beautiful medieval cities to explore ideas about the Healthy City and ways in which the project might usefully develop (see Box 8.2).

The initial atmosphere was one of excitement and energy but it was not to be without tension. On the very first day it transpired that local government elections the previous week had completely changed the political landscape. The Socialist Party, whose initiative Healthy Cities had been in Lisbon, had been displaced by a party from the political right. The last thing the new administration wanted was for the old regime to bask in the glory of a new WHO initiative and the organizing committee was made to feel anything but welcome.

I had been tasked by Ilona with producing a vision piece based on a personal sense of how my own city of Liverpool might reinvent itself by the year 2000. Having burned the midnight oil and dug deep into my creative juices in preparation, I found myself cut off in midstream of my delivery of 'Esmedune 2000:Vision or Dream? (A Healthy Liverpool)', by a hostile local chairwoman. The hard lesson we all learned from this early foray into local politics was that if Healthy Cities was to fly and to endure it would need to be owned across political party divides. In the event the Lisbon experience failed to stop the project from taking off.

Subsequently, further meetings in Gothenburg in October 1986 and in Barcelona in March 1987 focused on urban strategies for health, and appropriate indicators of the healthy city. The initially modest intentions for a four- to six-city project had to be changed to accommodate the enormous interest in the

Box 8.2 List of participating cities at the Lisbon Conference, 1986

Vienna	Turku	Dalby
Graz	Pecs	Stockholm
Brussels	Amsterdam	Aarau
Sofia	Rotterdam	Windisch
Horsens	Utrecht	Liverpool
Bremen	Warsaw	London
Hamburg	Lisbon	Manchester
Kassel	Barcelona	Oxford
Stuttgart	Granada	Swansea
Helsinki	Madrid	Belgrade

initiative. Following the first invitation to cities to apply for inclusion as WHO Project Cities, 11 cities paved the way and by 1988, 24 European Project Cities were involved together with as many as 100 other European cities in national networks and networks in Canada, Australia, and New Zealand. In addition some areas, notably the Valencia region of Spain, spontaneously developed their own extensive initiatives based on the WHO project.

For the next two years I was engaged in a hectic round of intensive workshops in cities across Europe, and increasingly further afield, working with extensive groups of citizens, professionals, bureaucrats, and city fathers and mothers with passion for their hometowns and the ability to make a difference (see Box 8.3).

The Healthy Cities Coordinating Centre in the Public Health Department at the University of Liverpool drew heavily on the good will and resources of the regional health authority to share and disseminate the growing number of stories of work inspired by the project, to support events, and for several years

Box 8.3 Healthy City Workshops, 1986–7

Holland	Denmark	Yugoslavia
Portugal	Austria	USA
Finland	France	Bulgaria
Canada	Germany	
Sweden	Spain	

to produce a widely distributed newsletter, 'Healthy Cities—Cities Fit to Live in', in emulation of the newsletter produced by the Health of Towns Association (See Figure 8.1).

In addition several European project cities each produced a documentary television programme for international transmission in conjunction with Channel 4 television of London. The first United Kingdom Healthy Cities conference was to be organized in Liverpool in 1988 and a further global conference with the British Council as sponsor in 1993.

By the time I stepped back from the European Project in 1988 to continue my work in the North West of England our team could reasonably claim that Ilona's original idea was well on its way to global dissemination and becoming part of an urban movement. Nor would I be able to detach myself so readily from the phenomenon of Healthy Cities. For years ahead I would be invited to help cities around the world to follow in the footsteps of the pioneering Europeans and later still, in 2016, I found myself back at the heart of things with Monika Kosinska now leading Healthy Cities into its seventh phase from the WHO office in Copenhagen.

The vision thing

The very framing of the WHO Project as 'Healthy Cities' proved to be energizing to large numbers of people but the first task was to stand back from what could be just a slogan and make it tangible so that it could lead to action. As we put it at the time, 'Healthy Cities is intended to take the Health For All Strategy off the shelves and into the streets of Europe' (2). What then were our visions of Healthy Cities?

The first brochure introducing the project to the world was produced in Liverpool with graphic artist Peter Jones. The genius of Peter's first work was to give us the basis of an archetypal city image which could be reworked to make it specific to cities around the world. The first brochure, produced in time for Lisbon, was an abstract representation. Within a short time it was succeeded by a second, more defined version which provided the template for cities to create their own images within a universal project.

The link between these two stages was an invitation to envisage how cities might be by the year 2000 and beyond. In the case of my own offering 'Esmedune 2000: Vision or Dream?', the starting point was the inspiration provided by William Morris's classic work from 1890, *News from Nowhere*. In his novel Morris's central figure falls asleep after attending a utopian political meeting and wakes up to find himself in a radically different future in which there is a proper balance between work, domestic life, and leisure and in which the arts

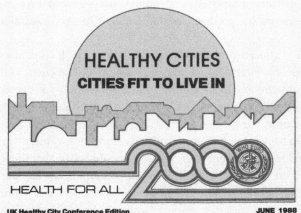

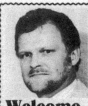

Welcome to Healthy Cities

WELCOME to the first edition of Healthy Cities, a newspaper which aims to assist people in developing the practice of the New Public Health in towns and cities around the world.

Healthy Cities Editor is Howard Seymour.

The last three years since the first European Healthy City Conference in Lisbon have seen a remarkable surge in support for the Healthy City concept.

During that time 24 cities have joined the WHO Europe Healthy City Project. However, these cities represent only a small proportion of the many towns and cities around Europe and across the world (most notably Canada and Australia) that are now involved. Healthy Cities has grown from a project to a movement which can involve — and be used by — all.

The idea of the Healthy City has been picked up suddenly because the time is right to plan for health in our cities, to introduce or re-introduce public health, and to move toward greater participation and involvement.

Becoming a Healthy City — a city fit to live in — is a popular and politically important decision. However, once this decision is taken we must move beyond the rhetoric and concentrate on making things happen. Action speaks louder than words.

What this newspaper aims to do is provide a forum for information exchange as well as provide readers with the opportunity to report the success stories, share contacts, swap ideas, list forthcoming conferences, report on projects and good practice, and anything else which may be pertinent to the Healthy Cities cause.

Healthy Cities aims to put people and cities in touch with each other.

If you have anything to report drop a line to: The Editor, Healthy Cities, Normanton Grange, Langham Avenue, Aigburth, Liverpool 17, England.

UK Healthy City Conference Edition **JUNE 1988**
An information exchange newspaper produced by the Healthy Cities Centre

Liverpool hosts major health conference

THE first ever United Kingdom Healthy Cities Conference was held in Liverpool at the end of March.

Although conceived as a United Kingdom conference, interest was world-wide with delegates attending from as far afield as Spain, France, Italy, the Netherlands, Yugoslavia, Denmark, Sweden, Canada and the United States.

The theme of the conference was partnership and the ultimate goal . . . to establish a movement which will measurably improve the health of city dwellers by the year 2000.

TOGETHER

A leading member of the organising committee Dr John Ashton said: 'We brought together towns and cities from every part of the United Kingdom and beyond to promote the idea of a new public health which goes far beyond the prevention and treatment of disease.

'The incidence of disease, sickness and premature death in our towns and cities is far too high and so we have to look at the contributory factors including unemployment, housing sanitation, food, water, general amenities, sport and recreation facilities, and transport.

'We are seeking to establish a movement which will strive to improve the general health of our citizens by improving the urban environment and conditions in the workplace. This will inevitably involve a greater liaison between all the people who can influence the factors which cause ill health; the doctors, health promotion experts and the city planners, to name but a few.'

Delegates at the three-day conference in Liverpool University heard from more than 30 speakers whose subjects ranged from medicine to architecture, employment to environmental

Continued Page 8

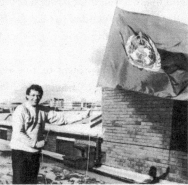

● *Dr John Ashton hoists the World Health flag on the final conference day.*

Figure 8.1 The 1988 Healthy Cities Conference Edition of 'Cities Fit to Live In'
Reproduced from Healthy Cities: Fit to live in. UK Healthy City Conference Edition. June 1988.
Copyright © Mersey Mirror Ltd.

play a full part in everybody's lives. Writing in Liverpool in 1986, when the city was facing possibly terminal decline, it was important to raise hope and point the way to a sustainable renaissance. The device I used was to frame a walk of discovery around the city in the year 2000, revealing a transformed New Age habitat, grounded in ecological principles, in which active citizens were able to live a full and democratic life without compromising the environment for future generations. At the heart of the new Liverpool were a set of philosophies, arrangements, and structures that reconciled the tensions it had inherited from dichotomies of the past:

◆ History/futures

◆ Art/science

◆ Male/female

◆ Technology/human relations

◆ Individual/social/

◆ Elitism/populism

◆ Reductionism/holistic

◆ Town/country.

The use of the name 'Esmedune' to describe the future city involved borrowing the Saxon name for the Toxteth area of the city where major riots had first drawn attention to a serious urban crisis. By using this old somewhat mysterious name that carried no baggage, it was intended to facilitate a fresh and optimistic approach to apparently intractable problems.

Agreement as to the precise nature of a healthy city is not necessarily easy to achieve. Certainly a healthy city is more than one which has good health services. My own use of dream imagery reflected a methodology that Trevor Hancock introduced to the project from work in Toronto. The thinking behind this approach is that although plans which take account of constraints are always necessary, to create a healthier future we must start with ideas and with a vision—those who start with 'realism' will never have a vision. William Morris's definition of health dating from 1884 resonates strongly not only with the underlying philosophy of Alma Ata and Health For All by the Year 2000 but also the core of Healthy Cities:

> At least I know this, that if a man is overworked in any degree he cannot enjoy the sort of health I am speaking of; nor can he if he is continually chained to one dull round of mechanical work, with no hope at the other end of it; nor if he lives in continual sordid anxiety for his livelihood; nor if he is ill-housed; nor if he is deprived of all enjoyment of the natural beauty of the world; nor if he has no amusement to quicken the flow of his spirits from time to time; all these things, which touch more or less directly on his bodily condition, are born of the claim I make to live in good health. (2)

Vision workshops based on the technique of guided dreams, with participants lying on the floor with eyes closed, imagining what they would find on return to their cities some years in the future, became an essential part of Healthy City workshops around Europe. They complemented a full day's programme in which typically up to 200 people, representative of all sectors, took part. Beginning with an intensive morning of lectures and discussions about the history and development of the New Public Health, the vision workshops bridged into an afternoon of thematic small group sessions covering such topics as housing, education, environment, lifestyles and leisure, work, transport, health and other public services, gender, and governance. Over lunch a separate briefing of politicians of all parties was held to create an awareness and acceptance of the ideas and proposals that might be heading their way. By the last session of the day a skeleton and an outline framework for developing a city health plan was the intended outcome, something to be fleshed out with wide public participation over the ensuing weeks and months. The energy liberated by many of these events was remarkable and the novel approach led to the sharing of a range of creative stories and approaches.

The idea of a healthy city incorporates the belief that the city is a place which shapes human possibility and experience and has a crucial part to play in determining the health of those living in it. According to Hancock and Duhl:

> a healthy city is continually creating and improving those physical and social environments and expanding those community resources which enable people to support each other in performing all functions of life and in developing themselves to their maximum potential. (3)

This carries with it the implication that in a healthy city there is some kind of agreed 'common gameboard', that, broadly speaking, people are pulling in the same direction; however, conflict and its resolution are also part of the healthy city. Yet each city is unique and has a life of its own, a soul, a spirit, even a personality; to understand a city it must be experienced as a complete entity and as a place for living. As the author and novelist Lawrence Durrell so elegantly expressed it:

> But as you get to know Europe slowly, tasting the wines, the cheeses and characters of the different countries you begin to realise that that the important determinant of any culture is after all—the spirit of place. Just as one particular vineyard will always give you a special wine with discernible characteristics so a Spain, an Italy, a Greece will always give you the same type of culture—will express itself through the human being just as it does through its wild flowers. (4)

At its most fundamental a city is unhealthy if it cannot provide its citizens with the basic necessities of life:

+ Safe and adequate food
+ A safe water supply
+ Shelter
+ Sanitation
+ Freedom from poverty and fear.

However, these alone are insufficient and most people expect much more, a range of environmental prerequisites, economic, physical, social, and cultural.

For most of recorded history cities have actually been unhealthy places in which to live, especially for their poorer citizens, and the implications in terms of inequalities in health and differential mortality rates are clear. It was in response to these problems that the Victorian public health movement came into existence and it is not by chance that town planning and public health have had such a close pedigree in the past.

It is perhaps not surprising that the awful conditions inspired thinkers to imagine urban utopias as a stimulus to change, nor that visions of the future should have influenced the town planner Ebenezer Howard, who developed the first 'garden city' suburbs in the United Kingdom at the end of the nineteenth century as a technical solution to the slums.

With the benefit of hindsight, many of the technical interventions of the latter part of the past century, such as housing estates and new towns, tower-blocks for the poor, and fully planned environments, are largely believed to have failed. Not only were people mostly not consulted and involved in deciding their own destinies, but one of their most precious assets for health—the networks of family and friends—was often negligently destroyed in the process. In creating a New Urban Public Health, it is necessary to move away from paternalism towards partnership and citizen control.

Core elements and tasks of the Healthy Cities Project

In taking inspiration from the work of the Health of Towns Association all those years before, what emerged from early discussions in the planning group was an initiative centred around five core elements:

1. The formulation of concepts leading to the adoption of city plans for health and wellbeing which were action-orientated and used Health For All and its targets based on health promotion principles as a framework.

2. The development of models of good practice representing a variety of entry points to action based on cities' own perceived priorities. These could range from major environmental interventions to programmes designed to support individual lifestyle change.

3. Monitoring and research into the effectiveness of models of good practice on health and cities.

4. Dissemination of ideas and experiences between collaborating cities and other interested cities.

5. Mutual support, collaboration and learning, and cultural exchange between the towns and cities of Europe.

The roadmap for achieving these objectives specified seven specific tasks that participating cities undertook to carry out as part of their responsibility to the project:

1. To establish a high-level, inter-sectoral group which brought together executive decision makers from the main agencies and organizations within the city. The purpose of this group was to take a strategic overview of health in the city and unlock their organizations to work together at every level.

2. To establish an inter-sectoral technical group as a shadow to the executive group to work on collaborative analysis and planning for health.

3. To carry out a community diagnosis down to the small area level, with an emphasis on inequalities in health and the integration of data from a variety of sources including the assessment of public perception of their communities and their personal health.

4. The establishment of sound working links between the city and the local institutions of education, both school and higher educational levels. These links were to not to be restricted to medical training establishments but were to include any department or institution with an interest in urban health-related phenomena. Part of this work would involve the identification of appropriate urban health indicators.

5. That all agencies would conduct a review of the health promotion potential of their activities and organizations. This should lead to the development of health impact statements making the health promotion potential in different policy areas explicit. It would include the recognition that within a city there are many untapped assets and resources for health, both human and material. In future years this would lead to the development of the WHO-supported work on 'Health in All Policies' and to an embrace of the work of John McKnight on asset-based community development (ABCD).

6. That cities would generate a great debate about health and wellbeing involving the public and working actively with the local media. This could include the generation of debate and dialogue using schools, community centres, museums, libraries, and art galleries. There was a recognition that

a city's own public health history provides a powerful focus for debate and learning. Part of this work is the development of effective health advocacy.

7. The adoption of specific interventions aimed at improving health and their monitoring and evaluation. The sharing of experience between cities and the development that underpins health, cultural links, and exchanges was seen as promoting a fundamental goal of the World Health Organization, the promotion of world peace and security.

The emphasis of these tasks was on developing enabling mechanisms which could be developed through healthy public policy, increased accountability, and public participation. It was also on breaking down vertical structures and barriers through partnership working. Buried away within the Healthy Cities initiative could be found many of the activities of the Health of Towns Association, bringing together key players in the cities, establishing a clear picture of health in different parts of the city, and developing advocacy and coalition building for change, intervention, and legislation.

Information and measurement

From the very beginning of the project the planning group attached great importance to work on indicators and measurement to demonstrate impact. Modern parameters appropriate for measuring the health of a city must span from such traditional and contemporary ones of environmental protection and the quality of the physical environment through measures of mortality, morbidity, and the quality of treatment and preventive medical services, into much 'softer' though equally important measures that define culture, participation, inter-sectoral collaboration, and levels of mutual support. In that early phase of the project much of the background thinking on indicators and measurement came from Trevor Hancock and Len Duhl. It also came from a set of papers provided for the Lisbon conference, and further meetings in Barcelona and Alicante in 1989 by Peter Flynn, a senior town planner with Liverpool City Council.

In setting the context, Flynn pointed out that 'the measurement of "health" in Britain has been dominated by two traditions of research. One focused on the relationship between health, and class or social status. The other has examined the geographical relationship between health and measures of income, poverty, or deprivation. The latter have been the basis for measuring the relative health of cities, and of different types of social areas within them' (5). Flynn used the example of small area analysis of health inequalities in Liverpool to illustrate the power of local data to galvanize political action. Using computer analyses of census and locally collected data, Liverpool City Planning Department had defined five standard data zones for the city which brought together spatially separate populations with shared characteristics such as income level and housing tenure type. It was clear from this that a further, social dimension of the WHO definition of health would be needed and that this would require development work and that the assessment of needs must be paralleled by assessments of assets and resources available.

An outline list of suggested indicators was drawn up as a result of workshops at the Lisbon meeting in 1986:

+ Demography
+ Quality of the physical environment including pollution, quality of the infrastructure, and housing
+ State of the local economy including unemployment levels
+ Quality of the social environment, including levels of psychosocial stress and quality of social support services, strength, and nature of local culture(s)
+ Personal safety
+ Aesthetics of the environment and quality of life
+ Appropriate education
+ Extent of community power and participation, structures of government
+ New health promotion indicators, e.g. participation in physical exercise, dietary habits, alcohol and tobacco use
+ Quality of health services
+ Traditional health indicators (mortality and morbidity)
+ Equity.

The description of the health of a city along these lines requires a multidisciplinary approach and a recognition of the validity of subjective data. In the context of an action plan in real time the approach to measurement also needs to be pragmatic; the observatory philosophy of 'good enough', rather than seeking a counsel of perfection sometime in the future is essential. What emerged from the discussions were the 'Barcelona Criteria' as a template for assessing suitable indicators of the healthy city:

+ That they should stimulate change by the nature of their political visibility and punch, through being sensitive to change in the short term, and being comparable between cities;
+ That they should be simple to collect, use, and understand, be either directly available at the time or available in a reasonable time at an acceptable cost; and
+ That they should be related to health promotion.

From the Alicante meeting came a preliminary list of measures for assessing progress towards achieving Health For All at the city level. Based on the Barcelona Criteria it included a variety of measures—holistic and analytic; subjective and objective; total population and target groups; determinants, action, and outcome; personal, community, and political; new and old—so as to give a broad overall impression of city health (see Box 8.4).

Tales and true stories; the beginnings of a movement

Healthy Cities projects did not begin with the Healthy Cities Project. The community gardens movement in North America is a good example of an ecologically orientated initiative arising from within communities and reflecting the philosophy of Health For All. In the socially stressed Regents Park area of Toronto local residents had combined with public bodies to produce a community garden managed by women from one of the tower blocks. This provided a focus for community integration, active recreation, a nutrition education programme, and the production of fresh vegetables by local residents on low incomes. In the South Bronx in New York, GLIE farms had responded to the growing interest in health foods by establishing a successful community business, growing and marketing fresh herbs to hotels and restaurants from a base in derelict industrial land within a community demoralized by unemployment and crime. Similar tales of urban regeneration were emerging from different parts of North America and were used to promote the growing momentum behind Healthy Cities. Other examples included Rails to Trails in the United States and Sustrans in the United Kingdom, community organizations which were actively converting disused railway tracks into cycling and walking routes.

The potential for allotment gardens, pocket handkerchief parks, small holdings, and animal husbandry in urban areas was identified as being significant as well as personal development programmes for teenagers such as 'Urban Adventures' and 'The Bronx Frontier', in New York. This was especially the case in towns and cities that had lost population and had an abundant supply of derelict land and unused buildings, assets just waiting for applied imagination. The social, psychological, physical, nutritional, economic, and environmental benefits of initiatives of this kind were increasingly becoming incorporated into the notion of the healthy city.

The importance of creating cities fit for children was well illustrated by the Seattle KIDSPLACE initiative. Faced with a familiar pattern of middle class flight from the centre of the city associated with fears for safety, Seattle found itself in a position where increasing numbers of people saw it as unsuitable to bring up children. The mayor commissioned a survey in association with a

Box 8.4 Parameters included in the WHO core list of the healthy city measures

1. Determinants

   Basic needs

       Shelter, housing, and homelessness

       Work and worklessness

       Income, poverty, and welfare

   Physical environment

       Air quality

       Accessibility

   Social environment

       Social support, loneliness, isolation

       Violence

       Work satisfaction

   Personal determinants

       Smoking

       Self-esteem

       Drunk driving

2. Action

   Political

   Community

   Personal

3. Outcome

   Perceived levels of health

   Restricted activity levels

   Perinatal health

   Mental health

   Food hygiene

   Coronary heart disease

   AIDS

4. Perception of the city

   Overall perception (proportion of people reporting the city as a good or very good place to live)

   Safety in the Neighbourhood (proportion of people reporting they feel safe walking at night in the neighbourhood).

local newspaper in which children were asked to identify how they felt about their city.

The children's responses were collated and used by the city planning department as the basis for a map of the city which represented the children's perspective and provided the basis for environmental and developmental action to create a more child-friendly city. In addition the children completing the survey were asked if they would like to be considered as a possible 'Mayor for the Day'. The young girl who was chosen said that her greatest concern was that when she was in a shop adults took precedence over children and that as mayor she would wish to do something about this. The outcome was window stickers for shops which proclaimed them as 'Kidsplaces' where children would be treated on an equal basis to adults and subsequently children began to be consulted on other matters concerning them.

The use of the KIDSPLACE approach was promoted by the Liverpool Healthy Cities Coordinating Centre and was picked up in Europe by Bremen, Kassel, Rotterdam, Turku, Barcelona, Liverpool, Oxford, and Horsens. In Barcelona, which was building up to host the Olympic Games in 1992, the Mayor Joan Clos, himself a public health physician, went further and involved the children of Barcelona in a highly participative summer-long initiative to plan the regeneration of the medieval area of the city and its connections both to the Olympic stadium and to the long neglected industrialized seaside area of the city.

Healthy Cities in Liverpool

The relationships that had been built up on New Public Health initiatives in Liverpool from the 1980s provided a good platform for developing Healthy Cities in the city. Following the Lisbon conference in 1986 I secured political support from all three major parties in the city. This was at a fraught time in the city's political history with an administration dominated by councillors in thrall to a Trotskyist view of social transformation. Consensual support for Liverpool to become involved with the WHO project was brokered by Councillor John Hamilton, a Quaker, socialist, and gentleman who was notionally the leader of the council at the time. The wisdom of this move is evidenced by Liverpool's continued involvement with WHO over 30 years later.

An immediate benefit from formal endorsement by the city was the access this gave to the expertise of city officers that kickstarted a focus on the pursuit of the core elements and key tasks as proposed by WHO and would lead quite quickly to a health plan for the city. This brought together the existing stories of recent public health work, not just by the local public health professionals on teenage pregnancy, drug-related harm reduction, and action on lifestyles, but also that which was community led. The example of the Eldonians achievements in urban regeneration and that of a group of women health activists, who campaigned successfully for the building of a local health centre, began to put flesh on the bones of the essence of Healthy Cities. Heavyweight support from the chairman of the regional health authority, Sir Donald Wilson, helped to mobilize other leaders of public, private, and voluntary sector bodies helped on by positive and creative relationships with the local media. Especially productive was an initiative to identify academics from across the city's universities who expressed an interest in working together on issues relating to the urban condition, to life and health. Almost 100 people came forward to take part in a series of workshops; town planners, architects, geographers, historians, social and health workers of various kinds, and social scientists as well as the usual suspects from public health. The initial output was an inventory of existing relevant research to Liverpool as a healthy city with a subsequent supplementary library of relevant student dissertation projects. This work spawned a number of interdisciplinary groups that continued to work together on supportive research and documentation for the city health plan (see Box 8.5)

Box 8.5 Liverpool Healthy Cities research inventory

- Ageing/the elderly
- Biological chemistry
- Child health
- Community studies
- Diet
- Education
- Health and regional economics
- Housing and urban regeneration
- Information systems and technology
- Land use
- Medical
- Pollution
- Public health history
- Social structures
- Sport and recreation
- Veterinary environmental health.

The early involvement of Liverpool as a WHO project city paved the way for a major conference which would facilitate the roll out of Healthy Cities both nationally and internationally.

The first United Kingdom Healthy Cities Conference, Liverpool 1988

The planning of the first United Kingdom Healthy Cities Conference took almost two years with sponsorship from a wide range of local and national bodies and businesses. It was immediately preceded by a two-day WHO workshop, 'Ecological Models For Healthy Cities planning', led by WHO environmental health expert Eric Giroult, a workshop which produced salient recommendations which were fed into the conference itself. Almost 500 delegates met in Liverpool University for a four-day smorgasbord of offerings by leading authorities on a comprehensive range of urban health issues.

In his conference introduction, Sir Donald Acheson reminded delegates that 'from the days of Jericho cities have been unhealthy places. Overcrowding, the accumulation of human excrement and waste, industrial effluents: each has brought its own category of disease. While at least in the developed world a great deal has been accomplished to secure within our cities adequate shelter; nutrition; heating; lighting; transport; work and education, even in these areas work remains to be done', before telling the conference that 'behaviour conducive to health and effective medical interventions even working together are not enough. Social and environmental policies which support health are also needed' (6).

The Liverpool conference achieved a remarkable level of media penetration with extensive coverage in the local and regional live and print media but also across the UK and beyond, including major broadsheet newspapers and broadcasters. This was as a result of the attention that was paid to reaching out to journalists and providing a professional level of facilities for them in the conference venue. It was also a reflection of the all-consuming interest that can be found in relation to our cities and the passions that they arouse. This has been a recurring theme of the Healthy Cities project since the beginning.

Principles of the ecological city

The WHO workshop on Ecological Models for Healthy Cities Planning, which preceded the Liverpool conference identified four important ecological principles that should apply to the overall planning of cities and to individual development proposals (6):

- Minimum intrusion into the natural state: 'The principle of minimum intrusion requires that new development and restructuring should reflect the topographic, hydrographic, vegetal and climatic environment in which it occurs. A close reference to the natural site will benefit drainage, ventilation, insulation, the indoor climate, the micro-climate and open and green spaces.'

- Maximum variety: 'Maximum variety should be aimed for in the physical, social and economic structure of the city. Land uses and activities should be mixed where this does not create hazards rather than separated and fragmented. A range of economic activities will make cities and communities less vulnerable to change and reduce social polarisation and inequalities.'

- As closed a system as possible: 'The principle of closed systems in urban and environmental health management would mean that waste is recycled within the urban area wherever possible and that water, energy and resources are renewable. The management of green spaces would maintain nature and recreational opportunities within cities.'

- An optimal balance between population and resources: 'Urban and population changes must relate to the fragile natural systems and environments that support them. Balance is required at the city and neighbourhood levels to provide a high quality and supportive physical environment, as well as economic and cultural opportunities' (6).

These principles are as relevant today as they were when they were first linked to the Healthy Cities project in 1988. One poignant irony of that workshop was that it included a presentation by Liverpool City Council engineers department on their approach to ensuring public safety in the local football stadia. Twelve months later 96 Liverpool football supporters would perish in the Hillsborough stadium disaster in Sheffield.

Healthy Cities, the wider picture; the project goes global

From the beginning there was a tension at the heart of the World Health Organization Project between the organizational need for a high profile public health intervention in Europe and the energy that was released by the project team promoting what turned out to be a contagious concept. In the event the project was to grow and develop well past the millennium under the inspired leadership of Ilona Kickbusch and administered after my initial establishment work by Agis Tsouros. The project evolved through six different phases until international health policy expert Monika Kosinska took charge after establishing the influential European Health Policy Alliance in Brussels. For over thirty years the WHO focus was contained within a framework of a finite number of cities in a contractual relationship based on the initial core principles and key tasks that had been outlined in 1986. Special interest groups around particular public health themes, working groups, and regular conferences enabled Europe-wide sharing of experiences and led to alliances across countries and between cities. One example of such work came from Gothenburg with the successful reduction in road accident mortality and morbidity by linking data from the hospital casualty department with that from the police; the ensuing intelligence was used in the city planning and engineers departments to put in place targeted changes in the road system in a more effective way than could be achieved by relying on death statistics alone.

From the early days cities took advantage of the new links to put on special events such as a summer camp of teenagers from participating cities that was held in Horsens in Denmark and the twinning of teen football clubs between Liverpool and Rennes in Brittany. The period of the late 1980s and early 1990s was marked by a deterioration in political stability in parts of Europe, in particular in the Balkans where public health leader Slobodan Lang was quick to see the value of mobilizing humanistic public opinion through the Healthy Cities European and other networks. At the 1988 conference in Zagreb, the challenge of putting on a major international event with almost no budget and a region sliding into civil war was met by mobilizing all the resources that human imagination could identify and deploy. Throughout the dark years of civil war in the former Yugoslavia, the Croatian Healthy Cities network continued to document the challenges to public health and drew support from colleagues across European cities, building on the legacy of regular summer schools that had brought people together in a search for peace and solidarity at the Inter-University Centre in Dubrovnik.

In parallel with the World Health Organization Project itself, other cities spontaneously began their own healthy city initiatives without waiting for WHO endorsement. Particularly impressive was the activity in the Valencia Region of Spain led by public health academics Concha Colomer and Carlos Alvarez with the active support of the region's medical director Joachim Colomer. In the Valencia region within a few short years over 80 per cent of the population was living in a local authority area that was part of the Valencia Healthy Cities network, giving significant momentum to the re-establishment of an effective public health movement in these post-Franco years.

Outside Europe, Greg Goldstein and his colleagues in the WHO office in Geneva promoted the Healthy Cities approach on a global scale with workshops and conferences in Alexandria and Tehran, Delhi and other Indian cities, Hong Kong, and cities in Australia and New Zealand.

In some parts of the world a focus on cities has been directly transferable whilst in others it has seemed more appropriate to frame interventions around towns, villages, or communities; more recently the language of 'place' has become commonplace. Having finished my time as Healthy Cities coordinator in Europe I had the privilege of facilitating the project's dissemination in many other countries. The approach had particular traction in South America and the Caribbean where it was adapted by Marilyn Rice from the Pan American Health Organization in Washington with an emphasis on healthy communities in the Americas, where elected mayors were able to provide highly visible leadership for public health. A highlight of this period was a conference in Medellin, Columbia in 1999 with 1000 elected mayors who had signed up with a commitment to implement a city health plan.

It was a mark of the momentum created by Healthy Cities and of the personal interest of Sir Donald Acheson that he was able to persuade his chief medical officer colleagues from around the world to choose rapid urbanization as the topic for technical discussion at the 1991 World Health Assembly where he would be chairman. I was privileged to be asked by Sir Donald to act as his rapporteur. These technical discussions take place prior to the political discussions where the outcome of the deliberations are received by health ministers; my task as rapporteur was to support the chairman and produce the outcome document which was made available overnight into the four WHO European languages (English, French, Russian, and German). Six background documents provided the meat for the discussions with a plenary session framed by contributions from the Director General of WHO, Dr Nakajima, and from three experienced Healthy Cities Proponents from different regions of the world.

The outcome of the General Assembly was a comprehensive set of recommendations which carried the force of World Health Organization formal policy making in relation to the following major areas:

◆ The prevention of excessive population growth with reference to balanced infrastructure, and rural and urban development;

◆ Strengthening urban development with regard to sustainability and health-supporting environments; cross-cutting policies in different sectors to promote healthy communities and environments; the development of suitable structures and processes for inter-sectoral and community participation;

◆ Appropriate decentralization of responsibilities for urban development and management;

- Reorientation and strengthening of urban health services to primary health care;
- Strengthening community participation and partnership working;
- Developing networks of cities and communities for health at the national and international levels; and
- Improving information and research for urban health.

The assembly went on to call for the community of international agencies to support these recommendations and for the WHO Director General to prioritize them. In a period of five years, Healthy Cities had gone from being a gleam in the eyes of that initial planning group to occupying a place at the heart of global public health attention.

From cities to settings and places

In the years since 1991, the focus on the city as a setting for health action has led to a range of other settings-based initiatives. The World Health Organization itself has promoted work on healthy schools and hospitals as well as healthy prisons, which led to another groundbreaking conference in Liverpool in 1995. Our continuing concern with behavioural and cultural aspects of public health and in particular of recreation spawned a set of initiatives including healthy nightlife focused on the night-time economy and healthy stadia based on the recognition that to reach men in particular it was necessary to engage with them in the settings which they naturally frequented (see Box 8.6). Both these initiatives have led to conferences which rotate internationally at regular intervals in common with the global conferences on 'harm reduction' which grew out of the Merseyside work on syringe exchange in 1986. In 1994, the Liverpool Public Health Observatory published a report on 'Health Care on Small Islands' for WHO Geneva, from where Greg Goldstein stimulated work in African countries on 'Healthy Market Places', whilst Martin White in Newcastle upon Tyne set about the creation of a 'healthy medical school', an example for higher education which was to lead to the publication of a report on the 'Health Promoting University' and the establishment of a 'Healthy Settings' unit at Central Lancashire University. Other productive outcomes included a network of European 'Regions For Health' led by Anna Ritsatakis from WHO Copenhagen, with initially six regions working together to share strategic approaches to the New Public Health.

These various streams of work, collaborations, and conversations in turn reinforced the growing interest in the application of health impact assessment and the later iterations of the idea of healthy public policy in the form of 'Health in All Policies'.

Following the interest generated by the original Merseyside Healthy Stadia Programme, a successful proposal was made to the European Commission in 2006 within the framework of the European Public Health Programme. The project worked initially with partner agencies in Finland, Greece, Italy, Latvia, Ireland, Poland, Spain, and the UK to develop the concept and suitable guidance. Subsequently the initiative has expanded significantly, is part funded by the World Heart Federation, works closely with the European Football Association, and has been prominent in UEFA's implementation of its tobacco-free stadia policy. Later work has focused on research to underpin the improvement in levels of physical activity and reduce sedentary time among football fans.

With the thirtieth anniversary of the launch of the WHO project and the end of its sixth phase, together with new leadership in the person of Monika Kosinska, by 2016–17 the time was right for a refresh and a review; part of this was to be a shift of emphasis from the idea of 'setting' to one of 'place', a concerted effort at securing prominent political leadership and the marriage of the aims of Healthy Cities to the Global Sustainable Development Goals as recently framed by the United Nations in 2015.

The relaunch of Healthy Cities in 2018 also coincided with the 40th anniversary of the transformational agenda set by the Alma Ata Declaration in 1977 and the spread of the European Healthy Cities Project to include Central Asia.

Box 8.6 Developing a European Healthy Stadia Network

The potential for using sports stadia as health-promoting settings began to be realized in the early years of the new century. One of the most significant developments in this field has been the formation of the 'European Healthy Stadia Network'. As a result of a number of regional initiatives in the North West of England, a working definition of a 'healthy' stadium was established in 2005, namely:

> Healthy Stadia are ... those which promote the health of visitors, fans, players, employees and the surrounding community ... places where people can go to have a positive healthy experience of playing or watching sport. (7)

Healthy Cities as places, local politicians, and the Sustainable Development Goals

The seventh phase of the WHO Healthy Cities project, launched in 2018, chose to refocus the terminology of the city as a 'setting' to that of 'place'. The argument was that ' "Place" transcends the physical environment alluded to by "Setting"—the buildings, streets, urban layout, and public and natural spaces, and includes social dimensions'. The use of the term 'place' implies a dynamic state of flux, an interaction between people with their biology and the physical, economic, and social environment. It is characterized by constant change, movement, and transformation that go beyond the physical setting and encompass the determinants of health and wellbeing. The social dimensions of 'place' include equity, inclusion, human rights, community resilience, empowerment, trust, ownership, the dynamics of human interaction, and the development of human and social capital. In proposing this new emphasis the Healthy Cities Project, together with its international networks, chose to position this new phase within a framework for action and a vision of the healthy city that included people, participating and thriving at levels of appropriate and attainable prosperity in a peaceful world without prejudicing the planet. At a workshop in Edinburgh in September 2017, in partnership with NHS, and Architecture and Design Scotland, a tool which had been developed and piloted in Scotland was tested by representatives of the European Healthy Cities networks and found to be valuable in taking forward the new phase. This 'Place Standard', with its 14 domains, offered a way of engaging with local people, professionals, and other stakeholders in assessing very different places and structuring conversations that could lead to change and progress (see Figure 8.2).

The shift from 'setting' to 'place' was also seen to be relevant to the transformative agenda of the United Nations 2030 Agenda and the Global Goals for Sustainable Development. As the parent body of the World Health Organization, the United Nations had been on a journey which had begun in Stockholm in 1972 with the UN Conference on the Human Environment and had led to the establishment of the World Commission on Environment and Development in 1983. It was the World Commission that had defined sustainable development as 'meeting the needs of the present without compromising the ability of future generations to meet their own needs', a definition which had provided the foundations of the first United Nations Conference on Environment and Development in Rio de Janeiro in 1992 and had resulted in what was to become known as 'Agenda 21' and in the year 2000, the Millennium Development Goals. Those goals were due to expire in 2015 and in the preparatory discussions it was decided to link new goals for development to sustainability. At the

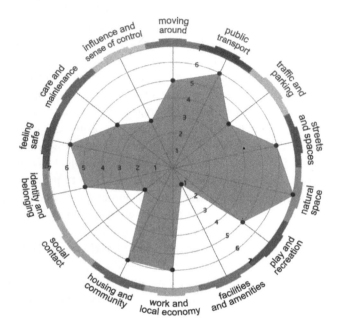

The Place Standard is a way of assessing places. Whether the place is well-established, undergoing change, or is still being planned, the tool can help you.

The Place Standard tool provides a simple framework to structure conversations about place. It allows you to think about the physical elements of a place (for example its open spaces and transport links) as well as the social aspects (for example whether people feel they have a say in decision making). Research shows that the way places function, look and feel can influence our health and wellbeing.

The tool provides prompts for discussions, allowing you to consider all the elements of a place in a methodical way. The tool pinpoints the assets of a place, as well as areas where a place could improve.

Figure 8.2 Place Standard—How good is our place?.
Reproduced from NHS Health Scotland. Place Standard. © Crown copyright 2017. Contains public sector information licensed under the Open Government Licence v3.0. Available at http://www.placestandard.scot/#/home.

Box 8.7 The United Nations Sustainable Development Goals

1. No poverty
2. Zero hunger
3. Good health and wellbeing
4. Quality education
5. Gender equality
6. Clean water and sanitation
7. Affordable and clean energy
8. Decent work and economic growth
9. Industry, innovation, and infrastructure
10. Reduced inequalities
11. Sustainable cities and communities
12. Responsible consumption and production
13. Climate action
14. Life below water
15. Life on land
16. Peace, justice, and strong institutions
17. Partnerships for the goals

Rio 20+ Conference a resolution, 'The future we want', was adopted by the UN member states and with it the new 17 goals and a total of 169 targets. Most, if not each, of these are directly relevant to the work of the Healthy Cities Project in the 2020s (see Box 8.7).

In making the connection between the continuing momentum of Healthy Cities and the United Nations ambitions for the year 2030, the political dimensions are clear and the role of local politicians and of civic leadership has come to the fore. A thousand elected mayors at a conference in Medellin in 1999 was an indication of what can be possible. Within Europe an important part of the sixth phase of the project was the establishment of a cross-Europe 'Summit of the Mayors'. With yet more echoes of the 'Health of Towns Association' of the 1840s historians will judge whether the twenty-first-century public health movement can match that of the nineteenth century. For myself, having been in at the conception of Healthy Cities in 1985 and its birth in 1986, it was a source of immense satisfaction to be still involved as it reached out into maturity to change the condition and the wellbeing of citizens around the world.

References

1. **Brundtland, G. H.** *Our Common Future: The Report of the World Commission on Environment and Development.* Oxford: Oxford University Press, 1987.
2. **Morris, William,** How we live and how we might live. Lecture given to the Hammersmith branch of the Socialist Democratic Foundation at Kelmscott House, 30 November 1884. Available at: https://www.marxists.org/archive/morris/works/1884/hwl/hwl.htm
3. **Hancock, T.,** and **Duhl, L. J.** Healthy cities: promoting health in the urban context. A background working paper for the Healthy Cities symposium, Portugal, 1986. Copenhagen: WHO, 1986.
4. **Durrell, Lawrence.** *Spirit of Place,* ed. **Alan G. Thomas.** Boston, MA: Da Capo Press, 1997.
5. **Flynn, P.** Health indicators: context and the next steps. A background paper for the Indicators meeting of the Healthy Cities Project, Barcelona, March 1987. Copenhagen/Liverpool: WHO, Liverpool City Planning Department, 1987.
6. **World Health Organization.** Ecological models for healthy cities planning. Report on WHO workshop, Liverpool, 25–27 March. Rapporteur P. Flynn. Copenhagen: WHO, 1988.
7. **Crabb, J.,** and **Ratinckx, L.** *The Healthy Stadia Programme Toolkit: Developing Sustainable Partnerships for Local Health Improvement Strategies.* A report for North West Public Health Team. London: Department of Health, UK, 2005.

Further Reading

Ashton, J. Esmedune 2000. *A Healthy Liverpool (Vision or Dream).* Liverpool: Department of Community Health, Liverpool University, 1988.

Ashton, J.(ed). *Healthy Cities.* Buckingham, UK: Open Universities Press, 1991.

Ashton, J., P. Grey, and **K. Barnard.** Healthy Cities—WHO's New Public health initiative. *Health Promotion* **1** (3) (1986), 319–23.

Ashton, J., and **J. Ubido.** The healthy city and the ecological idea. Paper presented at the Society for the Social History of Medicine. *Social History of Medicine* **4**(1) (1991): 173–81.

Barnard, K. *Lisbon Healthy Cities Symposium: Notes of Closing Address on Behalf of the Planning Group.* Copenhagen: WHO, 1986.

Beyond Health Care. Proceedings of a working conference on healthy public policy. *Canadian Journal of Public Health* **76** (suppl.) (1985), 1–104.

Brundtland, G. H. *Our Common Future: The Report of the World Commission on Environment and Development.* Oxford: Oxford University Press, 1987.

Duhl, Leonard J. (ed). *The Urban Condition. People and Policy in the Metropolis.* New York: Simon and Schuster, 1963.

Duhl, L. J. The healthy city: its function and its future. *Health Promotion* **1** (1986), 55–60.

Flynn, P. Health indicators: context and the next steps. A background paper for the Indicators meeting of the Healthy Cities Project, Barcelona, March 1987. Copenhagen: WHO/Liverpool: Liverpool City Planning Department, 1987.

Garcia, Pilar, and Mark McCarthy. Measuring Health: A Step in the Development of City Health Profiles. Copenhagen: World Health Organization Regional Office for Europe, 1996.

Hancock, T. Lalonde and beyond: looking back at 'A New Perspective on the Health of Canadians'. *Health Promotion* **1**(1) (1986), 93–100.

Hancock, T. Healthy Toronto—a vision of a healthy city. In *Healthy Cities—Concepts and Visions: A Resource for the WHO Healthy Cities Project*. Liverpool: Department of Community Health, Liverpool University, 1988.

Hancock, T., and L. J. Duhl. Healthy Cities: promoting health in the urban context. A background working paper for the Healthy Cities symposium, Portugal, 1986. Copenhagen: WHO, 1986.

Kilfoyle, Mary, and Mark Bellis. Club health: the health of the clubbing nation. Report of the First International Conference on Club Health, Liverpool, 1997.

Knight, L., and J. Ashton. Proceedings of the First United Kingdom Healthy Cities Conference, Liverpool, March 28–30, 1988. Published by Department of Public Health, University of Liverpool, 1990.

Liverpool City Planning Department. *Social Area Study: The Results in Brief*. Liverpool: City Planning Department, 1984.

Liverpool City Planning Department. *Inequalities in Health in Liverpool*. Liverpool: City Planning Department, 1986.

Lynch, Kevin. *Good City Form*. Cambridge, MA: MIT Press, 1981.

Mayor's Survey. KIDSPLACE—technical report. Seattle, WA, 1984.

Nunez, Agapito, Concha Colomer, Rosana Peiro, and Carlos Alvarez-Dardet. The Valencian Community Healthy Cities Network: assessment of the implementation process. *Health Promotion International* **9**(3) (1994), 189–97.

Squires, Neil, and Judith Strobl. Healthy prisons: a vision for the future. Report of the First International Conference on Healthy Prisons, Liverpool 24–27 March. Published by the University of Liverpool with the World Health Organization, 1996.

Tsouros, Agis D. (ed.). *Twenty Steps for Developing a Healthy Cities Project*. Copenhagen: World Health Organization Regional Office for Europe, 1992.

World Health Organization. *Alma Ata. Primary Health Care*. Geneva: WHO, 1978.

World Health Organization. Healthy Cities—action strategies for health promotion. First Project Brochure. Copenhagen: WHO, 1986.

World Health Organization. Background papers to Healthy Cities meetings in Goteborg and Barcelona. Copenhagen: WHO, 1987.

World Health Organization. The Healthy Cities Project: A Proposed Framework for City Reports. Discussion Paper for the WHO Healthy Cities Symposium Düsseldorf, June 1987. Copenhagen: WHO, 1987.

World Health Organization. Ecological models for healthy cities planning. Report on WHO workshop, Liverpool, 25–7 March. Rapporteur P. Flynn. Copenhagen: WHO, 1988.

World Health Organization. *European Charter on Environment and Health.* Copenhagen: WHO, 1989.

World Health Organization. The urban health crisis: strategies for health for all in the face of rapid urbanisation. Report of the Technical Discussions at the Forty-Fourth World Health Assembly. Geneva: WHO, 1993.

World Health Organization. City health profiles: how to report on health in your city. Copenhagen: World Health Organization Regional Office for Europe, 1995.

World Health Organization. City health profiles. A review of progress. Copenhagen: World Health Organization Regional Office for Europe, 1998.

Chapter 9

Culture, arts, and wellbeing

So hope for a great sea change
On the far side of revenge
Believe that a farther shore
Is reachable from here
Believe in miracles
and cures and healing wells.
Seamus Heaney, Nobel Laureate,

The Cure at Troy (1)

When, in 2010, the city of Derry/Londonderry in Northern Ireland was chosen as the first United Kingdom City of Culture, the Nobel-prizewinning Irish poet Seamus Heaney captured the hopes of many in the province and around the world. The 'Troubles' in Northern Ireland had begun in the late 1960s, were deeply rooted in the United Kingdom's colonial past, and had led to thousands of violent deaths before the 1998 Good Friday Agreement. This started a peace process which slowly brought about a reconciliation between the deeply divided communities. Derry/Londonderry had been at the very epicentre of the hatred between Catholics and Protestants and the decision to entrust the two communities with the stewardship of the first UK City of Culture was regarded by many as both foolhardy and high-risk strategy. In the event Heaney's hopes were more than fulfilled as previously sworn enemies came together to deliver an effervescent cultural programme that transcended the cultural divide and left a legacy of growing trust and security.

Hatred and violence remain a major threat to public health, one which requires all the creative and organized efforts of society to address.

In today's troubled world the various forms of artistic and cultural expression can offer a means to find common ground and pave the way to peaceful futures of mutual security. They also have an important part to play in the search for meaning which lies at the heart of what it means to be human and which is the foundation of our health and wellbeing.

My own awakening to the importance of culture and the arts in public health work began in the classroom at the London School of Hygiene and Tropical Medicine when our lecturer, Sidney Chave, had used three photographs, as a data set, to demonstrate the changing health status over time of London school children. Nor was Sidney's creative initiative, in theming two London public houses to explain the work of public health pioneer John Snow and social reformer Jeremy Bentham to ordinary citizens lost on myself or my classmates. On returning to Liverpool in 1982 I became immersed in work to generate a momentum for a new public health movement.

As this work shaped up, the need for an eclectic approach which recognized the value of connecting to cultural influences and drawing on the arts soon became apparent.

The Liverpool International Garden Festival, 1984

The first real opportunity to move the new way of thinking onto a larger canvas had come in 1984 with the International Garden Festival in Liverpool. The origins of the garden festival lay in the inner city riots which had afflicted Liverpool in 1981 and the economic crisis facing the city. Conservative Member of Parliament Michael Heseltine had been designated 'Minister for Merseyside' by the Prime Minister. Heseltine had proposed an International Garden Festival, on European lines, as a means to address several issues simultaneously: as a rationale for investing heavily in, and restoring, a large area of derelict docklands to pleasant and productive use; as a way of creating a new vision for Liverpool; and as a way to provide a platform from which the city could recreate itself economically and socially. In retrospect, this initiative, together with the later cultural programme in 2008 when Liverpool was European City of Culture, were strategic punctuation marks on the city's journey back from the brink of terminal decline.

The International Garden festival ran from April to October and would ultimately host over four million visitors. It seemed to provide the ideal setting for a holistic approach to the New Public Health.

Extensive discussions took place with the landscape architects and designers about how the site could be inseminated with a health perspective. One discussion was about the tides of the River Mersey and the Bidston Observatory on the adjacent Wirral Peninsular which generated the tide tables for mariners worldwide; how an interpretation of this might give people insight into a large-scale human habitat called 'Liverpool', its origins and reasons for being.

Another discussion centred on the use of the festival to explore the gulf between town and country, urban and rural, and their interdependence, addressing the fracture of understanding of city dwellers from nature, its rhythms, cycles, and seasons which had done so much to impoverish the lives of people living in the city. Although this ambition for the festival was tempered by practical realities it nevertheless produced a comprehensive range of initiatives in addition to the largest static health fair that had been staged until then.

Health was a major theme throughout the festival and was explored using music and dance, yoga, drama, and poetry together with static displays, such as in the area devoted to the growing of vegetables. There was extensive coverage in the live and print media both locally and internationally. The inclusion of long-term unemployed young people as health promotion assistants drew attention of the reservoir of untapped assets at a time of pessimism and fatalism.

The partnership with Liverpool poet and artist Adrian Henri

It was at this time that I first met the celebrated local poet and artist Adrian Henri, an encounter that would lead to a collaboration lasting almost 20 years until Adrian's death in 2002. As somebody who had always been drawn as much to the arts and humanities as to the sciences, I had been intrigued by C. P. Snow's thesis that science and the arts were becoming two cultures to the detriment of us all. Later, on a visit to the Exploratorium in San Francisco, I was to learn of the efforts that others had made to bridge the divide. Nuclear physicist, and a member of the group whose work had led to the invention of the atomic bomb, Frank Oppenheimer became disillusioned with the use to which his work had been put at the end of the Second World War, and had sought a change of direction. In establishing the Exploratorium as the world's first hands-on, interactive science museum, Oppenheimer's philosophy was that if science was to benefit humankind it must be interpreted through the humanities. To that end he developed a programme of artists-in-residence through which to promote a holistic approach to scientific education beginning in childhood.

My own efforts to maintain links with the humanities while studying medicine had been less than fruitful, with overtures to the arts world tending to fall on stony ground. All that changed when I met Adrian after my return to Liverpool in the early 1980s. As a teenager I had known of Adrian and his fellow Liverpool poets, Brian Patten and Roger McGough, who had achieved international fame following the publication of their anthology, *The Mersey Sound*, in 1967. The immediacy, humour, and down-to-earth contemporary relevance to 'baby boomers' navigating the heady excitement of being a teenager in the decade 'that sex was discovered' placed their work apart from the dry memories of school English literature. From the moment I met Adrian, through his contributions to our programme at the International Garden Festival, I found a generous and kindred spirit eager to explore the use of his gifts to see and interpret the world and support my ambitions for work in public health. In addition to his talents as a poet and artist, Adrian was a passionate educator with regular commitments in schools and colleges. This would lead to his becoming a feature on the Liverpool Masters in Public Health programme where an introduction to environmental, performance, and fine art would take its place alongside the quantitative and qualitative sciences and the history of public health.

The initial point of shared interest grew out of the environmental ideas running through the Garden Festival activities. In 1974 Adrian had published his book *Environments and Happenings*, which chronicled the tradition of works of art and of events which draw on environmental awareness to reach insights that can transcend consciousness. Typical of the humour evoked by some of the happenings described was the event in which wreaths were laid by mourners in Victorian dress at the site of demolished landmarks (e.g. a popular chip shop). The thinking behind the holistic approach to the garden festival was much influenced by this constellation of art and happenings connected to environment and particularly by some of the things that were going on in the neighbourhood adjacent to Adrian's house in the centre of Liverpool. Next to the nearby 'Cracke' pub, in an area notoriously 'demi-monde', with street prostitution and drug dealing, local community activist Lenny Cruikshank had established a small city farm, and took over the Second World War bombsite next to the Cracke to create a 'seaside for the day' for local children with sand provided by a local builder.

Following the Garden Festival, Adrian's involvement with public health education was a natural next step, an opportunity to link Sidney Chave's ideas with wider opportunities as we developed health promotion and sought public engagement. Adrian's subsequent work with Healthy Cities became ubiquitous as he spoke and made presentations at a number of conferences and workshops and provided commissioned poems. Adrian crafted the poem 'City 2000' in support of WHO's Healthy Cities and together with his partner Catherine Marcangeli created their own visual interpretation of my vision piece 'Esmedune', as a mural, a trompe d'oeil on a seminar room wall in the university department of public health (see Box 9.1, Figure 9.1). Over time 'Esmedune' also attracted the attentions of architect Rob Macdonald, who illustrated it in publication form with cartoons, and local students from Liverpool John Moores University who produced an animation version as part of their final exam coursework. It was

Box 9.1 'City 2000', Adrian Henri, 1986

In this city
filled with the sound of alarm-bells
police sirens howl
like animals mating.
Vagrants huddle together
in cardboard cities;
in a damp bed sit,
a girl dreams visions of Patmos
Cool, white spaces
The dust gleam of an ikon
The night
written in dripping white
on a railway wall
'Swarming city, city full of dreams'
In this city
the sound of the bulldozer is banished from the land
Swingeing custodial sentences imposed
on anyone designing a building finished in shuttered concrete
Car parks burst into flower
narcissi, blue flags, lilies-of-the-valley
pushing up through the tarmac,
the streets heaped with yellow marigolds
All planning decisions are referred to
The postman Ferdinand Cheval
Charles Rennie Mackintosh
and
Antoni Gaudi
(all speaking through a medium)

The city
no longer an embarrassment,
The too-much loved mother
at the school speech day
lipstick blurred
smelling of gin-and-lime
As the sun rises over this city
Your morning face on the pillow
Through strands of dark brown hair

> **Box 9.1 'City 2000', Adrian Henri, 1986** (*continued*)
>
> The river lying back open to the day
> the lace curtains of terraced houses
> Sing like schoolchildren.
>
> This city
> is your mother
> and your lover.
>
> She is your first thought
> and your last.
>
> She is your future and your past. (2)

Adrian's distinctive voice that provided the soundtrack to the acclaimed and powerful short film produced for the 1988 Healthy Cities conference in Liverpool.

Adrian Henri's humanistic drive and empathy was to be in evidence under the extreme challenge of the Hillsborough football stadium disaster of 1989. He gave voice, through his poetry, to many thousands of football supporters and their families in the form of a poem, 'The Bell', which he wrote in solidarity with the bereaved (see Box 9.2).

Adrian's poignant canvas *Flowers for Liverpool*, which captured the unique Liverpool mourning for those killed, in the form of floral tributes on the Kop

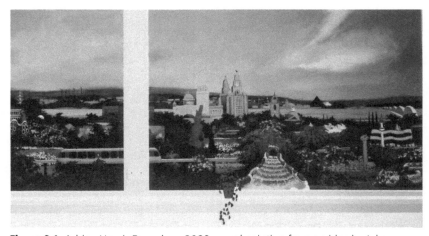

Figure 9.1 Adrian Henri, *Esmedune 2000*, mural painting from an idea by John Ashton. Department of Public Health, University of Liverpool.

Box 9.2 'The Bell', Adrian Henri, April 1989

The bell
tolled all afternoon
we did not send to ask
for whom.
It told of flowers
heaped in a goalmouth,
red and blue scarves
heaped together at an altar;
it told of
eyes like TV screens
haunted by last night's images,
tears dried by the April wind.
As the flags at half-mast
stirred overhead
the deep bell
still toiled in our heads
long after the light had gone. (3)

terraces, is to be found on the wall at Anfield, the home of Liverpool Football Club (see Figure 9.2).

In 1990, sponsored by the British Council and building on Liverpool's collaboration with Healthy Cities in Spain, Adrian participated in the Fallas celebrations in Valencia, giving poetry readings and speaking at events about the role of environmental art and happenings in Healthy Cities. The Fallas is a remarkable traditional cultural event dating back to the Middle Ages and involving the whole community. Each neighbourhood works throughout the year to produce topical sculptures known as Fallas, the children producing their own smaller versions. Each Falla, loaded with fireworks, is burned during a city-wide, 5-day-long street party known as La Crema. In his reflections on the relevance of such environmental and performance art to public health Adrian identified a range of possibilities. During the 1980s with the threat of HIV/AIDS looming, the new 'plague' was among the themes to be picked up in the 'Ninos', or sculptures.

Celebrating 150 years of public health in Liverpool

In 1997 we marked the 150th anniversary of the appointment of William Henry Duncan as Medical Officer of Health in Liverpool with a programme of events

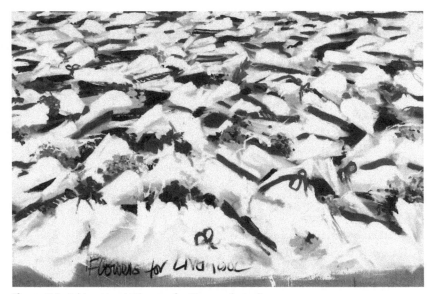

Figure 9.2 Adrian Henri, *Flowers for Liverpool*, acrylic on canvas.
Reproduced with permission from Adrian Henri's estate. Copyright © Adrian Henri Estate.

to celebrate and commemorate the public health achievements which had begun with Duncan. Working in partnership with the health authority, the city council, and the voluntary sector and community, a small team consisting of Maggi Morris from public health, together with public health historian Sally Sheard, organized and curated a programme of over 100 events to run throughout the year. Pride of place went to the use of the visual and performance arts, music, and public lectures to raise awareness of Liverpool's rich public health history and its relevance to contemporary challenges. Re-enactments of sentinel public health moments were staged with actors including the passing of the 'Liverpool Sanitary Act' (in Liverpool Town Hall) and the inaugural meeting of the Liverpool Health of Towns Association (in the original music hall building). A procession of public health professionals, accompanied an actor playing Dr Duncan, visited sites of key public health significance in the city.

An updated edition of the book *The Pool of Life: A Public Health Walk in Liverpool* was published to commemorate the year's celebrations (see Figure 9.3).

A centrepiece of the year's activities was the appointment of Adrian Henri as 'Public Health Artist-in-Residence' for the year. Adrian convened a group of some 16 fine and installation artists who were challenged to respond through their work to the idea of what public health means to the public, professionals, and communities. The artists were chosen not only for the quality of their work but also for the range and variety, styles and media which they could deploy. The result was 'The Dr Duncan Art Show', wrapped around an existing special

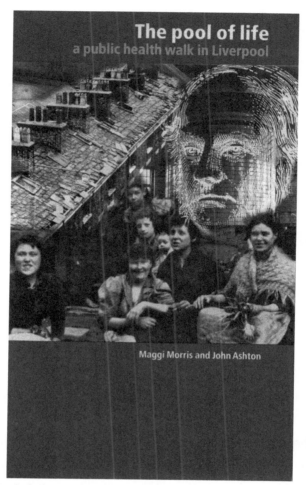

Figure 9.3 Pool of Life: A public health walk in Liverpool.
Reproduced with permission from Maggi Morris and John Ashton.

exhibition including full-scale facsimiles of slum housing and sanitation in the city's Museum of Liverpool Life. Called 'A Healthy Place to Live', the exhibition explored 150 years of public health themes, focusing on current and future challenges. Adrian believed that there was a public assumption about artists being self-indulgent and living in ivory towers. He felt that with the focus of the exhibition and art show on realism it could help to dispel that image with artists engaging with real and wider social issues (see Figure 9.4).

The 150th anniversary celebrations left a permanent legacy in the form of the Duncan Society, a forum for the multidisciplinary and public discussion of health-related issues.

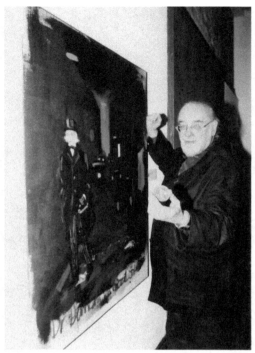

Figure 9.4 Artist Adrian Henri with his canvas Dr Duncan in Seel Street, acrylic on canvas, during The Doctor Duncan Art Show.
Reproduced with permission from Adrian Henri's estate. Copyright © Adrian Henri Estate.

Public health, culture, and the arts: the wider agenda

The eclectic range of activities developed during the 1980s and 1990s reflected back to an earlier tradition of public health being fully engaged with the worlds of town planning, architecture, art, and design. The Healthy Cities initiative itself had made play of the close relationship between public health and town planning in the nineteenth century. The involvement of leading architects in the design of pioneering health centre buildings in the twentieth century has already been referred to and our own work in Liverpool had brought us into collaboration with architects working at the community level to bring about public engagement in the design of buildings which they would use. More generally, alongside the evolution of the new public health thinking, there was a growing interest in the use of art in medical and clinical settings.

Initially, the involvement of the arts in clinical settings was quite narrow, took the form of artwork on the walls of hospitals and health centres, and was dependent on local interest or on finding a local champion; for example, patients waking up from surgery in the recovery suite at Liverpool's Royal Infirmary would find themselves surrounded by Adrian Henri's murals of Monet's gardens at Giverny in France. This was still far away from the situation in parts of Spain where a set percentage of capital budgets for public buildings was earmarked for public art. The potential scope for greater ambition was promoted at Manchester Metropolitan University, initially by Peter Senior and later by Clive Parkinson. I was fortunate in being able to develop a collaboration with them, initially through teaching in Manchester, later through more systematic initiatives.

Following the 2001 organ retention scandal at the Alder Hey Children's Hospital in Liverpool it was proposed to the hospital management that one way to rebuild trust with its public would be through an arts and health programme. It was felt that this had the potential to facilitate public engagement that might transcend the trading of past hurts. The outcome was a remarkable initiative, championed by a senior clinician, which went well beyond 'art on walls' to embrace the live and performing arts together with novel forms of humanistic therapy appropriate to a young patient group.

At this time too, I was fortunate in being able to build on the emerging track record of work in this field to persuade the government-sponsored North West Arts Council to co-fund the production of a regional strategy for arts and public health which was drawn up by a talented young arts entrepreneur, Polly Moseley. In turn this spawned a region-wide network of arts and health initiatives supported by Manchester Metropolitan University.

This provided the base from which to secure 'invest to save' funding from the government treasury to support this work across the local National Health Services. Later, in Cumbria, it was possible to move the agenda even further by engaging with asset-based community development (ABCD), following visits from John McKnight to the county. John led workshops which were attended by many of those active in the world of arts and health. Subsequently, a vibrant event was held which explored the implication of ABCD for arts and health. One of the main tenets of ABCD is that everybody has gifts, that people and communities are 'half full, not half empty'; the role of real education is to discover, and reveal those gifts, in contrast to a professional model which seeks to fix things from outside and can create dependency undermining personal agency.

As the arts and health movement matures, it should develop this philosophy of facilitating and enabling the flourishing of popular participation.

The role of storytelling in public health

The power of narrative in achieving transformational change has been understood since biblical times, the Old Testament being full of parables illustrating the contemporary health beliefs of the time. For most children 'Once upon a time' will be among their earliest memories.

Whilst the story of John Snow and the Broad Street pump has probably been part of most new students' introduction to public health, too often a diet of dry statistics is the extent of the offer to health authorities, public bodies, and worst of all to the general public. Although we now live in a world of scientific orthodoxy we also live in a world where so-called 'fake news' has been able to literally 'Trump' evidence-based facts in the public domain. Whilst statistics may be 'people with the tears wiped off', to quote Major Greenwood of the London School of Hygiene and Tropical Medicine, data and intelligence are no longer sufficient to win arguments for public health. For that, something else is needed. That something else leads us down the path to cultural and artistic expression and not least storytelling.

Culture and the arts in public health: the example of dementia

The modern epidemic of dementia can in some ways be compared with the challenge posed by cholera to our Victorian predecessors.

Although the underlying biological causes of the range of conditions associated with deteriorating brain function are an important focus for research and hopefully intervention in the future, environmental and social considerations form part of a complete understanding and response. This new challenge needs to be met by the organized efforts of society. Cultural activities and artistic attention must inevitably be part of this as we struggle to make sense of this bewildering condition.

An example of how the cultural sector can contribute directly to ameliorating the impact of dementia not only to those suffering from the condition but also in support of families and carers has come from the National Museums of Liverpool, where I had the privilege of being a board member. 'House of Memories' is a museum-led dementia awareness programme in partnership with the local mental health trust, Mersey Care.

The programme offers training, and access to resources and artefacts and museum-based activities to enable carers to provide person-centred care for people living with dementia. It works by sharing memories with people living with dementia, improving communication, and focusing on the person rather than on the condition. The evaluation of this novel intervention found that, overwhelmingly, participants reported that the training increased their awareness and understanding of dementia and helped them to see those living with the condition differently and to respond more effectively. In parallel with this work in Liverpool, architects Bill Halsall and Rob Macdonald, who had long been involved at the interface between design, the built environment, health, and wellbeing led an inclusive process with other professionals, dementia sufferers, and their carers to produce a two-volume manual for architects. *Design for Dementia—A Guide* brought together academic and experiential knowledge in one place to facilitate best practice in building design, to enable dementia sufferers to continue with quality life despite their condition. From cradle to grave, in all aspects of life's journey, cultural and artistic expression helps us to make sense of our short span and can contribute to our health and wellbeing (See box 9.3 and Figure 9.5).

Box 9.3 From 'A Dream of Doctor Duncan', Adrian Henri, 1997

'... this Duncan
Hath borne his faculties so meek, hath been
So clear in his great efforts, that his virtues
Will plead like angels....'

—Shakespeare, *Macbeth*

As I was a-walking down Paradise Street
a figure in black I happened to meet
a smile on his face instead of a frown
a ghost walks the streets in Liverpool Town

He presses his nose to the window
to see rows of whirling glass eyes
in the brightlit launderette
like a child at christmas.

Choking cellars of Cazneau Street,
Dark courts of Duke street . . .

Turning on impulse to home, he walks down Seel Street;
dazed by the neon lure of nightclubs,
he does not notice the familiar figures
huddled on the steps of the Mission of Charity.

Cheapside and Lace Street,
Blind alleyways of Milton Street . . .

He nods approvingly at grids and litterbins,
tuts to himself as he notes cracked pavements,
burst-open black bags, polystyrene food-trays,
drifts of chip-papers, abandoned copies of THE BIG ISSUE.

Effluent-filled entries of Edge Hill
Dark empire of the Necropolis . . .

Tracing his daily route from Rodney Street
to work in Upper Parliament Street
he sees the girls' white familiar faces at the corner,
wonders only at the shortness of their skirts.

Guiding Star, Garrick, Clare Wheeler
Ghost plague-ships haunt the Mersey mist . . .

He smiles at the curtained glow of tidy houses
where typhoid and cholera once stalked the street,
does not see the bleak estates where skeletons dance
to the electric beat of poverty.

As I was a-walking down Paradise Street
a figure in black I happened to meet
a smile on his face instead of a frown
a ghost walks the streets of Liverpool Town.

Joined by the crinolined shade of Kitty Wilkinson,
he pauses politely to offer an arm.
Beyond the traffic lights their figures fade
in the Grimshaw mist of the Old Dock Road (4).

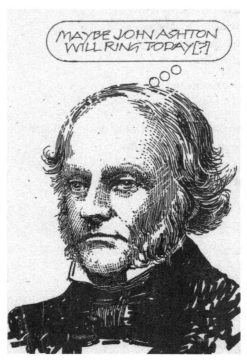

Figure 9.5 Cartoon of Dr Duncan by Fred O'Brien.
Reproduced courtesy of Louise O'Brien.

References

1. **Heaney, Seamus.** *The Cure at Troy: Sophocles Philoctetes.* London: Faber Drama (2018).
2. **Henri, Adrian.** City 2000. Commissioned poem for Liverpool Healthy Cities (1986). Cited in Ashton, J. R., The death of an artist: Adrian Henri, 1932–2000, *Journal of Epidemiology and Community Health 56*(1) (2002), 72–5.
3. **Henri, Adrian.** The Bell, in *Liverpool Accents: Seven Poets and a City: An Anthology.* Liverpool: Liverpool University Press, 1996.
4. **Henri, Adrian.** A dream of Doctor Duncan. Commissioned poem for 150 years of public health in Liverpool (1997). Cited in Ashton, J. R., The death of an artist: Adrian Henri, 1932–2000, *Journal of Epidemiology and Community Health 56*(1) (2002), 72–5.

Further Reading

Ashton, John. Let's invest in real health. *Create, A journal on the value of art and culture,* 91–6. Arts Council England, 2015.

Halsall, Bill, and **Rob MacDonald.** *Design for Dementia* (2 vols). Halsall Liverpool: Lloyd Partnership, 2016.

Henri, Adrian. *Environments and Happenings.* London: Thames and Hudson, 1974.

Henri, Adrian. *Paintings, 1953–1998.* Liverpool: National Museums and Galleries of Merseyside/The Bluecoat Press, 2000.

Morris, Maggi, and **John Ashton.** *The Pool of Life: A Public Health walk in Liverpool.* Liverpool: The Bluecoat Press, 2007.

Parkinson, Clive, and **Mike White.** Inequalities, the arts and public health: towards an international conversation. *Arts and Health 5*(3) (2013), 177–89.

Senior, Peter, and **Jonathan Croall.** *Helping to Heal: Arts in Health Care.* London: Calouste Gulbenkian Foundation, 1993.

Seymour, Howard, John Ashton, and **Peter Edwards.** Health museums or theme parks: a new approach to intersectoral collaboration. *Health Promotion 1*(3) (1986), 311–17.

Sherman, Barry. *Cities Fit to Live In: Themes and Variations A to Z.* London: Channel 4, 1998.

Snow, Charles Percy. (1959). *The Two Cultures.* London: Cambridge University Press, 2001.

Chapter 10

Reflections

Sitting at my desk to describe the challenges, joys, and frustrations of 40-plus years in the public health frontline, at a time of such great change, has been both nostalgic and poignant. Most occupations become quite routine after the first flush of novelty has past, even with the most esoteric specialism. To be a generalist, such as a director or consultant in public health, not knowing what the next challenge will be, is a privilege. To be a good generalist is arguably more difficult than to be a good specialist. I hope that I have captured a flavour of the joy and satisfaction to be found and the personal resourcefulness necessary to serve the people in protecting and improving health at the population level.

In paying tribute to those giants whose shoulders contemporary practitioners stand upon, we are brought face to face with dynamic and rapidly unfolding situations, constantly evolving and in flux. They demand a response, often in an incomplete state of knowledge. 'It would be prudent' to do 'such and such', even when the evidence base is thin, is something that never deterred John Snow from his classic intervention in Broad Street in 1854. Nor is a shortage of resources an acceptable response when faced with dire threats to whole neighbourhoods, cities, or countries. William Henry Duncan's response to Edwin Chadwick, that the establishment of public health in Liverpool, in the 1840s, consisted of himself, did not prevent him from mobilizing the citizens and the town's assets to ensure that the disaster of cholera in 1848 was not repeated six years later. The timescale of these distant events assumes an elasticity when the stories are laid out end to end and in some kind of sequence. I find it startling to consider that my grandmother, Agnes, was born in Daulby Street in the centre of Liverpool only 40 years after Duncan and Snow were walking their public health beats, the same length of time as my own career. From cholera and the workhouse via the Boer War and two world wars, to a totally different world of globalization with an agenda of the multiple pathologies of longevity and of mental ill-health, almost within living memory.

As a child of the welfare state, I entered the world when a new public health era was still to dawn. The demographic transition with its shift from infectious to non-infectious disease was just beginning to impact on health policy with ramifications that are being felt with the domination of hospital medicine over prevention and primary health care. We were to learn the hard way with the appearance of new, serious infectious, diseases that nature has many more tricks up its sleeve; as ecological science has matured we have begun to understand the importance of working with nature rather than seeking to impose our will on it.

As part of that privileged cohort that came of professional age in the 1960s and 1970s we were blessed with constant gifts of wisdom and support from the wartime generation that had returned from battlefields and pre-war economic miseries determined to build a new Jerusalem. Many of our teachers saw the route map as including a public health highway, and despite the new and emergent agenda they recognized the importance of lessons from history. I make no apology for my deference to the staff at the London School of Hygiene and Tropical Medicine, and in particular to Sidney Chave, whose insights have informed my own efforts to contribute to this noble cause. It is worth repeating them here: serendipity, plagiarism, independence, intelligence, coalition-building, resourcefulness and pragmatism, humanitarianism and moral tone, communication, mobilization, multidisciplinary team leadership, sustainable organizations, a galvanizing idea, and the need for public, political, and professional education. I hope the importance and relevance of each of these has been done justice in this book.

The work we began in England's North West in the 1980s started with a community diagnosis and evolved from there. By having a big picture in place, and political support from the right quarters, it was possible over time to be not only strategic but also pragmatic. A key part of the capacity building that followed was the launch of a new Masters in Public Health in the University of Liverpool based on the Alma Ata Declaration, and the WHO Strategy of Health for All by the Year 2000. In the course of time a regional focus was able to shape a series of complementary courses in universities across the North West to produce something approaching a virtual regional school of public health in the form of an academic network, an idea which was then picked up nationally. The success of these initiatives can be judged by their impact on producing local, regional, and national public health leaders, many of whom had passed through the Liverpool and North West training system. The reputation of the region in public health and its ability to respond to challenge continues to be high.

The thinking behind the original Public Health Observatory in Liverpool was persuasive and led to the roll out of regional observatories across the country, providing useful and timely intelligence to the local and regional system. It is a matter of regret that, after the ill-conceived health service reforms in 2013 and the creation of Public Health England, centralizing tendencies came to the fore and the new agency saw fit to drop the Observatory name. This pre-occupation with the national level demonstrated an ignorance of history and in particular the original vision of John Simon. This outcome was but one manifestation of the recurrent obsession with health service structures led by short-term thinking.

These weaknesses with their tendency to undermine coherent action and robust pursuit of the mission of public health were not confined to the statutory bodies. In some countries such as Canada, the United States, and Australia, national public health associations provide highly visible and loudly heard voices for public health advocacy. During the 1990s we established a North West Public Health Association in the North West with some success. With the establishment of a national association, the North West PHA was folded into it and for some ten years there was a highly effective counterweight to institutional inertia with an annual conference exceeding 1000 delegates. Over-dependence on grant aid from government and the failure to build a mass membership led to its demise together with the rise of managerialism in public health and a desire by government and its agencies to control the agenda. Nor were other membership organizations immune to the insidious influence of government and its related bodies. As President of the Faculty of Public Health of the UK Royal Colleges of Physicians, for three years from 2013 to 2016, I tried my best to go beyond the restrictive covenant of overseeing the acquisition of professional standards. Rather I tried to develop a meaningful independent voice for public health in the United Kingdom, a 'must go to' source for journalists and the media and a trusted voice. This did not sit comfortably with the managerial ethic so strongly held by many of the faculty officers, despite it being part of the original vision of the faculty's founders, and it was an uphill struggle. It remains to be seen whether a professional college with its craft interests and desire for proximity to power can ever be an independent force for disruptive change and progress. Similarly, it is an open question whether a public agency, as close to government as Public Health England, can ever do justice to the public need for that autonomous and trusted voice prepared to take the fight for health to all its enemies, including the vested interests of commerce. At the time of writing the promise is not good. The road is littered with past agencies, including the Health Education Council, the Health Education Agency, and the Health Protection Agency, which were closed down when they attempted to rise to the occasion. In the case of Public Health England, it has preferred to stay on the comfortable side of buttered bread. The jury is still out on its value.

When I set off to medical school in Newcastle upon Tyne, over 50 years ago, public health was out of fashion and what was left of it was narrowly medical. I was fortunate in my choice of university because it had always been grounded in its community and the flame of public health was kept burning long enough to inspire many of us to sign up. We have had some wonderful times and been able to witness and contribute to the never-ending story that is public health. Having been in at the conception of the WHO Healthy Cities Project and still being around as it reaches maturity, I can testify that even an organization as managerially top heavy as the WHO can be creative and relevant. With the continuing domination of our British public health institutions by technical and managerial fetish, at the expense of creativity and social mobilization, the prospects do not currently look good. It is my hope that this account of one person's journey, an eyewitness to the New Public Health, can engage and provide direction and support to the millennials who are now picking up the baton. The prize is the Health of the Public, 'The Highest Law'.

John Ashton
Liverpool and Dent, September 2019

Index